Clinical Skills for the Ophthalmic Examination

Basic Procedures

Second Edition

Lindy DuBois, MEd, MMSc, CO, COMT

Emory Eye Center

Atlanta, Georgia

Series Editors:

Janice K. Ledford • Ken Daniels • Robert Campbell

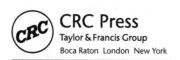

CRC Press

Taylor & Francis Group

Boca Raton London New York

CRC Press is an imprint of the
Taylor & Francis Group, an **informa** business

First published in 2006 by SLACK Incorporated

Published 2024 by CRC Press
2385 NW Executive Center Drive, Suite 320, Boca Raton FL 33431

and by CRC Press
4 Park Square, Milton Park, Abingdon, Oxon, OX14 4RN

CRC Press is an imprint of Taylor & Francis Group, LLC

Library of Congress Cataloging-in-Publication Data

DuBois, Lindy, 1948-
  Clinical skills for the ophthalmic examination : basic procedures /
Lindy DuBois. -- 2nd ed.
    p. ; cm. -- (Basic bookshelf for eyecare professionals)
  Rev. ed. of: Basic procedures. c1998.
  Includes bibliographical references and index.
  ISBN-13: 9781556427497 (alk. paper)
  1. Ophthalmic assistants. 2. Eye--Diseases--Diagnosis.   I. DuBois,
Lindy, 1948-   . Basic procedures. II. Title. III. Series.
  [DNLM: 1. Diagnostic Techniques, Ophthalmological. 2. Ophthalmic
Assistants.   WW 141 D815c 2006]
  RE72.5.D83 2006
  617.7'154--dc22

                                        2005020149

ISBN: 9781556427497 (pbk)
ISBN: 9781003523185 (ebk)

DOI: 10.1201/9781003523185

Dedication, First Edition

To my lifelong support system, Ethel, Don, Ellen, Doni, and Don, Jr., with love and gratitude.

Dedication, Second Edition

To my partner in life, Keith Lindsay - Thank you for the love, support, and respect.

Contents

Acknowledgments

I was honored to have been asked to contribute to this series. In thinking about the individuals who helped get me to the point where I could even consider undertaking such a task, I have to begin with my mother, Ethel, who instilled and encouraged my love of the written word. I was most fortunate to have been guided through my ophthalmology training by Barbara Cassin, an unconventional, open-minded, dedicated teacher who provided some remarkable opportunities for her students. My hopscotch career has given me diverse experiences in clinical ophthalmology and the most wonderful circle of friends and colleagues (too numerous to name, but you know who you are! Special thanks to Alfredo and Steve for jump-starting my publishing career). Many thanks to editor Jan Ledford for her kind words, encouragement, and gentle persuasion. Some of the work on this book was supported by the Emory Eye Center; I am most privileged to be working there (thank you, Mary) among a world-class faculty and staff.

Lindy DuBois, MEd, MMSc, CO, COMT

About the Author

Lindy DuBois is a certified ophthalmic medical technologist (COMT) and certified orthoptist (CO). After college, she worked as a chemist at the University of Florida and then undertook her ophthalmology training there. During this time, she also began work on her master's degree in health occupations education. Since finishing her training, Ms. DuBois has been on the faculty of ophthalmic technology training programs at the University of Florida in Gainesville, the University of Southern California in Los Angeles, and is currently the assistant program director in the master of medical science in ophthalmic technology program at Emory University in Atlanta, Ga. She received her MMSc from Emory in 1994. In addition to her teaching duties, she has worked in university clinics as well as private practice and has been the clinical coordinator of numerous clinical research trials.

Ms. DuBois has taught numerous courses and presented many papers for professional organizations, academic programs, and community groups. In addition to scientific publications, she has authored or reviewed sections of the home study course published by the American Academy of Ophthalmology and chapters in *Fundamentals for Ophthalmic Technical Personnel*. Ms. DuBois feels fortunate to have found her niche in this, her second, career. She is a cheerleader for the profession—encouraging and supporting entry into and advancement in the world of eyecare.

Introduction

Working in the field of medicine is immensely rewarding when the desire to serve is combined with the knowledge and skill to do so. The specialty of eyecare provides unsurpassed opportunities for job satisfaction and professional advancement. Most people value sight above all our other senses. As assistants, the work we do to help preserve and refine vision brings obvious joy to our patients. Perhaps, though, the role we play in dealing with patients who have lost vision is even more important because it requires not only technical knowledge, but also compassionate and ethical treatment.

It is a challenge to efficiently gather accurate information about a person's visual status. We have to know what questions to ask. We have to know what tests to perform and in what order. We have to know how to use and maintain an ever-expanding array of instruments. We must cultivate a kind and respectful "chairside" manner. This book is meant to teach the most common tests performed in the office. In addition, there are sections on how to obtain an accurate history from the patient, what is expected of you if you assist in minor surgery, and what you should know about common ocular medications. Because the assistant often has the first and most contact with the patient, I have emphasized the care and handling of the people who need our services.

I hope this book gives you the tools to be a skilled and efficient ophthalmic or optometric assistant. I also hope you will be stimulated and encouraged to go beyond what has been offered here and seek a deeper knowledge. The more the patient understands his or her condition or treatment, the more he or she becomes a partner in medical care. The more you know, the more you can do to help your patients achieve their visual potential.

Lindy DuBois, MEd, MMSc, CO, COMT

The Study Icons

The *Basic Bookshelf for Eyecare Professionals* is quality educational material designed for professionals in all branches of eyecare. Because so many of you want to expand your careers, we have made a special effort to include information needed for certification exams. When these study icons appear in the margin of a *Series* book, it is your cue that the material next to the icon (which may be a paragraph or an entire section) is listed as a criteria for a certification examination. Please use this key to identify the appropriate icon:

Opt   paraoptometric

OptA   paraoptometric assistant

OptT   paraoptometric technician

OphA   ophthalmic assistant

OphT   ophthalmic technician

OphMT   ophthalmic medical technologist

Srg   ophthalmic surgical assisting subspecialty

CL   contact lens registry

Optn   opticianry

RA   retinal angiographer

Chapter 1

Preliminaries: History, Exam Strategy, and Office Drugs

KEY POINTS

- Treat every patient with respect.

- Always protect the patient's privacy and preserve confidentiality.

- A complete and accurate history is the foundation of the examination.

- An examination strategy will streamline data collection and lessen test contamination.

The Patient

Patients seeking medical treatment may be fearful or anxious about their office visit. The ophthalmic or optometric assistant is usually the patient's first contact in the clinical setting; therefore, he or she should try to establish a rapport with the patient. A positive first impression will set the tone for the whole visit. This includes minimizing the patient's wait time as much as possible.

It is of greatest importance that every patient be treated with respect and kindness. For example, adults should not be addressed by their first names unless they request it. It is helpful to remember that each patient is not just a professional client but a person who represents our most important source of job satisfaction. The eyecare professional should treat each patient as if he or she were a special visitor: putting him or her at ease, explaining procedures, giving clear instructions, empathizing, and inspiring confidence.

Every patient exam requires some preparation, attention to detail, and attention to the patient. Some patients require more intensive professional and personal attention than others. Regardless of a patient's personal status (whether physical, emotional, or social), every person deserves respectful, caring treatment. There is no typical patient; each patient brings unique problems and needs to the visit and must be treated as an individual. In addition to technical skills and knowledge, the assistant must bring compassion to the exam. Some special problems include accommodating patients who are 1) elderly; 2) visually, mentally, or physically impaired; 3) non-English speaking; 4) illiterate; or 5) very young.

The assistant should remember to help elderly patients who have trouble with mobility and allow a reasonable amount of time to listen to the patient's medical complaint. The assistant needs to be attentive and patient during the examination without sacrificing efficiency. For example, a casual external examination of the patient can be done while the patient describes the problem.

Helping the visually impaired can sometimes be frustrating. Never assume that the patient wants or needs assistance. Simply ask the patient if he or she would like help. This shows respect for the person's ability to care for him- or herself. However, once a need for help is established, there are a few things the eyecare professional can do to allow the patient to feel confident while maneuvering through the office. First, make sure obstacles have been moved out of the way and that other office personnel are aware of the need for a clear path. When walking, the patient should grasp the leader's bent arm at the elbow. The leader should hold his or her own upper arm against the body, thereby holding the patient's fingers or hand between the body and arm so that the patient is walking slightly behind and can feel the leader's body as it changes direction. The leader should never "tow" the patient by the hand; the patient will not feel confident that he or she will not run into walls or door jambs. (Try both ways with a friend whose eyes are closed and notice the difference in control of the "patient.") Once the patient is ready to be seated, turn him or her so that the backs of the legs are against the seat of the chair and place the patient's hands on the arms of the chair. During the exam, the assistant should guide the patient's head or chin onto the chin rest, being careful to inform the patient before making physical contact.

Mentally and physically impaired patients should be assisted as necessary. A mentally impaired patient will almost always be accompanied by a caretaker. The caretaker should stay with the patient at all times to help with the history and assist in completing the ocular exam. A mentally impaired person should never be forced to cooperate, because this may cause anxiety and agitation, preventing the completion of the exam. If it becomes impossible to continue the exam, the assistant can inform the doctor and allow the patient to calm down in another (non-exam) room. A note can be made in the patient's chart that he or she was noncompliant.

Physically impaired patients may require help maneuvering into the exam room and then into the chair. When a patient is in a wheelchair, it should be rolled close to the exam chair, and the brakes on each wheel should be set before the patient begins the transfer. The eyecare professional must be careful not to injure him- or herself while assisting the patient and should ask for help from other office personnel or those accompanying the patient. Again, the patient can determine how much assistance is needed. It is often useful to have the doctor come to the patient rather than having to move the patient again.

Language barriers are often difficult to overcome during an ocular exam because so much depends on the patient's responses. At the time the appointment is made, if the patient does not speak English, he or she should be instructed to bring someone who can translate. This is also true for hearing impaired patients who use sign language. If no translator is available, the history will be fragmented, and instructions to the patient probably will not be understood. However, the patient can still be taught the "Tumbling E" test for acuity, and most other tests do not require a response (ie, are *not* subjective). Illiterate patients can also be tested this way.

Infants and young children present a special challenge because they are often shy or afraid and may be reluctant or unable to verbally communicate. While questioning parents, the professional should not ignore the child. Infants will respond to the examiner's smile and touch. Ask parents of infants returning to the office to postpone feeding the child and to bring a bottle to the visit; a hungry baby taking his or her bottle will not be so disturbed by the exam. Younger children can be gently questioned during the conversation with their parents; they will feel less threatened if they are made part of the process. Older children and teenagers should be treated with the same respect as adults, but a more casual attitude may help these patients feel more comfortable.

In addition to good communication skills, the eyecare professional should be attentive to the patient's comfort, expectations, and especially to the patient's right to privacy. A happy, compliant patient is one who is made to feel that he or she is a partner in the medical team.

Confidentiality

One of the most important aspects of the interaction between the patient and *any* health care worker is the issue of privacy. The very nature of providing good health care requires that the provider know personal medical and social information about the patient. This information is considered strictly confidential and may not be divulged by anyone with privileged access to it without the patient's consent. The health care worker must treat *all* patient information with equal respect for privacy; the patient is the only person who can decide which information might be damaging or embarrassing. In addition to not discussing privileged information outside the office, the health care worker must also be careful not to talk about a patient in the office hallways, where other patients might overhear the conversation.

The Health Insurance Portability and Accountability Act (HIPAA) was passed in 1996 to ensure the continuity of a person's health insurance coverage and to protect a person's health information. The latter goal has become the primary focus of HIPAA, and medical providers must now obtain a patient's consent for disclosure of protected health information (PHI) that is not for the express purpose of claims payment or continued care or treatment.

What the Patient Needs to Know

- You have the right to privacy.

- The information you give is kept in confidence.

- You have the right to be treated with respect.

History

Getting a complete and accurate history of a patient's ocular, medical, and social conditions may take more time than the actual eye exam. A good interviewer develops the history with focused and careful questioning, allowing the patient time to tell the story while directing the conversation with pointed questions. After the introductions, the first question to the patient is to elicit the chief complaint: "Are you having a particular problem with your eyes or is this a routine check-up?"

Another reason for recording a thorough history is that different billing codes require specific history categories or numbers of items within categories. Since the billing code is not assigned until the end of the visit, it is important to cover as much information as possible so that the physician can make an unrestricted choice of codes.

Chief Complaint

The patient is asked for the primary reason for the visit and a description of the problem. The chief complaint should be written (in abbreviated fashion using key phrases) on the medical record in the patient's own words, if possible. The chief complaint should be a concise statement of symptoms, onset, duration, and cause of the problem, if known.

In particular, the physician needs to know what signs (things that are observable by another person) and/or symptoms (things only noticed subjectively by the patient) are present and what has been the course of their onset. The history of this particular problem, often called the *history of present illness* (HPI), is then detailed by asking when the problem began, whether it is chronic or intermittent, whether it is progressive, and whether its onset or development are associated with any other events (such as ocular injury or contact lens wear problems). The HPI should also include the course of any previous similar episodes and the results of diagnostic tests and/or medical or surgical treatment.

If this information is being elicited because the patient called in for an unscheduled appointment, the patient will go through a screening and classification process, or *triage*, to determine the urgency of the visit. An *emergency* requires immediate attention, sometimes beginning before the patient comes to the office (eg, irrigating an eye with a chemical injury). An *urgent* situation requires attention within 24 to 48 hours, and *routine* problems are those that are minor or have existed for some time and may be addressed within a week or so. Each practice should have guidelines for determining the time frame for seeing patients with various problems.

Past Ocular History

Patient questioning logically progresses to determine any prior ocular problems. The technician should ask about the refractive history: does the patient wear optical correction, when was the first prescription, and what has been the frequency of prescription changes? The patient should also be asked about prior eye infections or injury, medical and/or surgical treatment (especially refractive surgery), and any adverse reactions to treatment. Chronic or recurrent ocular inflammation may have been investigated for associated systemic illness (such as lupus or arthritis), and the patient should be questioned regarding a diagnostic workup and both ocular and systemic treatment. If the patient wears contact lenses, the technician should determine the type (hard or soft), the wearing time and comfort, and especially the disinfection regimen.

Partially sighted or blind patients should be asked about the circumstances of their visual loss, but it is equally important to determine if quality of life is being enhanced by visual and/or mobility aids and whether the patient has adequate information regarding support agencies.

Past Medical History

The patient's medical/surgical history is best elicited by asking closed-ended questions such as, "Do you have any medical problems such as high blood pressure, diabetes, heart disease, or arthritis?" If the patient answers, "Yes," a history of each disorder should include onset, duration, and treatment. If the answer is "No," a more open-ended question may be asked: "Have you ever had any other disease or serious illness that required treatment or hospitalization?" The same strategy can be used to determine surgical history: first asking about common operations such as appendectomy, hysterectomy, or thyroidectomy, then following up with questions about the outcome of the operations or any complications. Whenever possible, the dates of all procedures should be documented.

Occasionally, it may be necessary to ask sensitive or possibly embarrassing questions, such as those regarding sexual medical history, HIV status, or pregnancy history. The technician should follow practice guidelines to decide whether to include these questions in taking the history or to defer them to the physician.

Family Medical History

The medical history of the immediate family (parents, siblings, and children of the patient) is important for the discovery of possible inherited disorders or heritable tendencies. The patient should be asked about the presence of any known ocular disorders in the family, such as glaucoma, high myopia, strabismus, or retinal degenerations. If the patient is not sure, ask if any family member must use prescription eye drops or has had any laser treatment or eye surgery.

If the patient has a known inherited disorder, it is useful to ask about any other family members or distant relatives who have similar diagnoses or symptoms. With this information, a "family tree" can be developed to show the inheritance pattern (eg, skips a generation or passed through the mother) and for use in genetic counseling.

The family medical history should cover the same major disorders as the patient's medical history. Questions should be asked regarding the incidence of diabetes, hypertension, cardiovascular disease, neurological disease, inflammatory disorders, etc.

Medications

Any medications prescribed by a physician must be listed and the dosages recorded. Eye medications must be listed with the eye in which they are used (right eye [OD], left eye [OS], or each eye [OU]) and, especially for glaucoma medications, the time they were last used. Many systemic medications may have an effect on the eye and on the patient's visual acuity and/or visual field.

Table 1-1
Common Prescription Abbreviations

q	every
qd	once daily
bid	twice daily (every 12 hours)
tid	3 times daily (every 8 hours)
qid	4 times daily (every 6 hours)
h	hour
q 2h	every 2 hours
hs	bedtime (hour of sleep)
soln	solution (drops)
ung	ointment
gtt	drop
mg	milligram
mcg	microgram
ml	milliliter

Diuretics, aspirin or other anticoagulants, and corticosteroids are among many systemic drugs that affect the physiology of the eye. It may also be important to know how long certain drugs have been used. Over-the-counter (OTC) medications and herbal and vitamin supplements may also be listed. The abbreviations for common dosages are listed in Table 1-1.

Allergies/Drug Reactions

It is very important to ask the patient if he or she has ever experienced any allergies or other types of reactions to medications. The medicine and type of reaction (hives, nausea, etc) should be documented. Drugs causing reactions should also be listed on the outside of the front cover of the chart to alert future examiners. Sulfa and the "-cillin" drugs, especially penicillin, are common sources of adverse reactions. It is important to ask about reactions to local anesthetics or fluorescein dye, since topical anesthetics and this dye are commonly used in ophthalmology. If the patient reports never having a drug reaction, the initials "NKDA" (no known drug allergy) may be written. Any other allergic reactions, such as contact dermatitis (tape, latex), chemical reactants (sprays, fumes), or food or environmental allergies (seafood, hay fever), should also be listed.

Interim History

When the patient is returning for a follow-up visit, a brief history of the patient's condition since his or her last visit will help direct the exam. The patient should be asked about any improvement in the problem for which he or she is being treated, including satisfaction with glasses prescribed at the last visit, if applicable. A dissatisfied patient will usually report this before being asked, so a sympathetic and helpful attitude on the part of the assistant will help defuse any anxiety or anger the patient may have. The patient should be asked about any new problems, diagnoses, medications, reactions, or treatment since the last visit. If the physician prescribed or changed medicines during the last visit, the assistant must determine if the patient has been using the medicines as prescribed (or if he or she has not been using them at all). Any other pertinent information offered by the patient should also be documented in the chart.

What the Patient Needs to Know

- Bring your medications to the visit.
- Bring all glasses you currently wear.
- Bring medical records if you have them.
- Report any allergies or reactions to medicine.

Exam Strategy

An efficient, accurate examination requires common sense as well as good technical skills. Efficiency begins before the patient enters the exam room. The medical record itself should be current, with exams listed consecutively and lab results or operative reports appropriately filed. Pertinent information from the prior visit(s) should be brought forward onto the day's work-up sheet only after verifying it verbally with the patient. The most recent exam is especially important in that it should contain any changes in medications prescribed or any instructions given by the doctor for the next (this) exam.

After the history has been taken, the eye examination is performed, beginning with visual acuity and including assessment of refractive error (retinoscopy and/or refractometry), lensometry, assessment of pupil function and ocular motility, slit lamp exam (biomicroscopy), measurement of intraocular pressure (tonometry), and evaluation of the retina (funduscopy), among others. By convention, the right eye is examined first, and the data are recorded accordingly. This practice helps avoid confusion and misremembering when both eyes have been examined before any data are written down. Each of these exam elements will be discussed in detail in later chapters.

The examination routine is similar in most general practices: the visual acuity at distance and near is determined first, followed by lensometry and/or keratometry. If refractometry is performed, it is done next, keeping both the patient's spectacle correction and keratometry readings in mind. The motility, pupil function, confrontation visual fields, and color vision tests may be performed next. Finally, the slit lamp exam and tonometry are done, followed by pupil dilation, if applicable. Of course, every procedure is not done at every visit. The exam can be tailored to individual patients, and a logical routine can improve efficiency. For example, all "glasses on" tests can be done together, or a casual external exam of the patient's face or eye position can be done while taking the history.

There are some tests that can contaminate or negatively affect the results of later tests. Whenever the examiner suspects a problem with binocular function (eg, convergence insufficiency or intermittent exotropia), all binocular tests must be performed before the patient undergoes tests requiring covering one eye; even the vision is not checked first in this case. This allows the patient to use whatever binocularity he or she does have without breaking fusion with the occluder. All tests of visual function, refractometry, and pupil function must be performed before the patient's pupils are dilated. Corneal sensation and reflex tearing must be tested before an anesthetic drop is placed in the eye. Evaluating the surface of the cornea should be done routinely before contact tonometry (applanation, Tonopen™, pneumotonometry) is done. Having a pre-examination "plan" in mind allows the examiner to list the tests to be done in an order that will keep one test from adversely affecting another.

Common Office Drugs

A wide variety of topical (drops or ointments) and systemic drugs (pills, injections, or syrups) are used in optometry and ophthalmology. These may be categorized as either *diagnostic* or *treatment* drugs. Diagnostic drugs are used to make a determination of the status of the eye; for instance, topical anesthetics are used to check the intraocular pressure, and dilating drops are used to evaluate the retina. Treatment, or therapeutic, medications are used to control or cure whatever disorder has been diagnosed (eg, drops used to control the intraocular pressure in glaucoma or antibiotics for an infection).

Diagnostic Drugs

Anesthetic Drugs

These are topical drops or sometimes injected drugs that numb the front surface of the eye. This procedure allows instruments such as the tonometer to be applied to the eye without causing patient discomfort. Other minor procedures such as gonioscopy, foreign body removal, and suture removal or adjustments also require the use of anesthetic drops. The most common anesthetics used in the office setting are proparacaine (Ophthaine™, Ophthetic™, Alcaine™, AK-Taine™) and tetracaine (Pontocaine™). Minor procedures may require other topical anesthetics that are longer-lasting or penetrate tissue more effectively (lidocaine, cocaine, procaine, mepivacaine, or bupivacaine).

Anesthetic medications, although commonly used in the clinical or surgical setting, are not benign. These drugs are very toxic to the corneal epithelium, and continuous use can cause erosions, ulcers, and eventually perforation of the cornea. There may also be systemic side effects. *Under no circumstances* should anesthetic drops be given to a patient to take home. The assistant should also be alert to the possibility that a patient with eye pain may take a bottle of anesthetic from the exam room.

Mydriatic (Dilating) and/or Cycloplegic Drugs

Dilating drops act on the iris dilator muscle to cause contraction or on the iris sphincter muscle to cause relaxation. Either action expands the pupil (mydriasis) and prevents the automatic pupillary constriction that occurs in bright illumination. This allows the use of instruments that provide a well-lit view of the inside of the eye. The common mydriatic agents are phenylephrine (Neo-Synephrine™), hydroxyamphetamine (Paredrine™), and epinephrine.

Cycloplegic drops also dilate the pupil. However, these drugs have the secondary function of paralyzing the ciliary muscle, thereby preventing accommodation (focus at near). This second function is particularly important in assessing the refractive error of children or of hyperopic (farsighted) adults. Cycloplegic refractometry provides a true assessment of the refractive error with the eye at rest. The cycloplegic drugs may last a few hours (tropicamide) to as long as 2 weeks (atropine). Tropicamide (Mydriacyl™) is the most common cycloplegic drug used in the office, but others include cyclopentolate (Cyclogyl™), homatropine, scopolamine, and atropine. Homatropine and scopolamine are more likely to be used to paralyze the ciliary muscle and iris sphincter to increase patient comfort in the case of intraocular inflammation. Atropine ointment may be used at home in children who will be returning to the office for a refractometry.

Table 1-2
Commonly Used Therapeutic Drugs (Brand Names)

Antibiotics

Polysporin	Tobrex	Vigamox
Polytrim	Ilotycin	Ak-sulf
Genoptic	Chloroptic	Sodium Sulamyd
Ocuflox	Ciloxan	Chibroxin
Zymar		

Antiviral

Vira-A		
Viroptic		

Antifungal

Natacyn		

Steroids

Pred Forte	Decadron	HMS
FML	Maxidex	Lotemax
Flarex	Vexol	Inflamase

NSAIDS

Ocufen	Acular	
Proteral		
Voltaren		

Diagnostic Stains or Dyes

Stains are often used in the office to show defects in the corneal epithelium and conjunctiva. Fluorescein, an orange solution, appears bright green against a blue background when viewed with cobalt blue filtered light. This dye demonstrates the loss of epithelial cells, such as that seen in a corneal ulcer, punctate keratopathy, or an abrasion. Fluorescein is used in combination with a topical anesthetic to perform Goldmann applanation tonometry. The dye may be provided on dry sterile paper strips or in an anesthetic solution (Fluress™, AK-Fluor™). There is the danger of *Pseudomonas* contamination of fluorescein solutions; this bacterium can cause a devastating ocular infection. Bacterial contamination is discouraged by the preservative in the solution.

Lissamine green and rose bengal are colored dyes that demonstrate degenerating epithelial cells on the surface of the cornea. These dyes are applied to the eye and viewed under white light at the slit lamp.

Therapeutic Drugs

Therapeutic drugs are used to treat ocular disorders such as infections, allergies, or glaucoma. Some of these drugs cure diseases, some are used to control the disease process, and some help to diminish the patient's symptoms. Although most drugs used for treatment are prescribed for the patient to use outside the office, some are administered in the office. It is important for the eyecare professional to be familiar with different classes of therapeutic drugs in order to obtain an accurate and complete history (Table 1-2).

Anti-Infective Drugs

Antibiotics

Antibacterial drugs may either destroy bacteria (*bactericidal*) or stop their reproduction (*bacteriostatic*). Different antibiotics are effective against different organisms. Some are very specific for a particular class of organisms; others are broad-spectrum (ie, effective against a wide variety of bacteria). Therefore, it is important to take cultures before treatment has begun. While the cultures are incubating, the patient can be started on a broad-spectrum medication and then later switched to a more specific drug, if indicated by the culture and sensitivity tests.

Topical antibiotics are most useful when ocular bacterial infections are limited to the cornea and conjunctiva. Deeper infections of the corneal stroma or interior eye require drugs that are capable of penetrating the outer corneal layers. When topically applied drugs are not effective, they can be administered in periocular, subconjunctival, or intravitreal injections. Some severe ocular infections may require systemic medication.

Patients should be instructed to adhere to the dosage regimen; prolonged use or overuse of antibiotics may lead to the development of bacteria that are resistant to the drug. In addition, because antibiotics also destroy the body's normal bacteria, prolonged use may promote the overgrowth of other disease-causing bacteria that are normally inhibited. Patients should be warned of the possibility of a reaction to the drug; this is usually limited to a local allergic or sensitivity reaction but may be more severe.

Antiviral Drugs

Antiviral drugs are used to treat infections caused by the herpes simplex virus (HSV) or herpes zoster virus (HZV). Topical drugs are often used alone when the viral infection is superficial. Anti-inflammatory and systemic antiviral drugs may be added when the infection is more severe.

Antifungal Drugs

Ocular infections caused by fungal organisms are less common than other infections but can have devastating effects on the cornea or intraocular structures. Microscopic fungi reside everywhere on plant material, so patients who present with a severe ocular infection must be questioned about trauma by tree or bush branches, wood particles, or other projectile plant material. Once a fungal infection has been confirmed by history or culture, antifungal medications are administered topically, subconjunctivally, intravitreally, or systemically.

Anti-Inflammatory/Anti-Allergic Drugs

Anti-inflammatory drugs may be classified as steroidal or nonsteroidal. Synthetic steroids are used for their strong anti-inflammatory properties. They are indicated for external or intraocular inflammation caused by allergies, infections, toxic reactions, or immune reactions (such as corneal graft rejection). They are also very effective against the intraocular inflammation associated with auto-immune disorders, such as rheumatoid arthritis or lupus, and may be administered topically, systemically, or by periocular injection. Steroids are powerful agents that may have serious side effects. They are immunosuppressive and affect the hormonal, skeletal, and muscular systems when administered systemically. Systemic steroids may also have extreme psychological effects or cause stomach bleeding. Topical ocular administration can cause glaucoma or cataracts. Because of their immunosuppressive properties, these drugs may allow the proliferation of infectious microorganisms. Steroid use cannot be stopped suddenly but must be discontinued slowly.

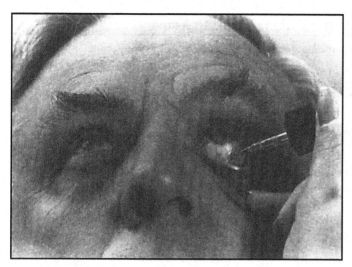

Figure 1-1. Instillation of drops. (Photo by Mark Arrigoni.) (Reprinted from Herrin MP. *Ophthalmic Examination and Basic Skills*. Thorofare, NJ: SLACK Incorporated; 1990.)

Nonsteroidal anti-inflammatory drugs (NSAIDS), although not usually as effective as steroids, may be used in milder cases of inflammation or at the end of a steroid taper. This class of drugs is extremely valuable clinically because it can have the desired anti-inflammatory effects without the negative side effects of steroid drugs.

A more detailed discussion of anti-infective and anti-inflammatory drugs, as well as anti-glaucoma drugs, may be found in the Series title *Ophthalmic Medications and Pharmacology.*

Instillation of Ocular Medication

Proper instillation of drops and ointments will ensure that adequate medication contacts the ocular surface and that contamination of the bottle or tube is minimized. Drops are instilled by gently pulling the lower lid away from the globe and allowing a drop to fall into the pocket created between the lid and the eye (Figure 1-1). Care must be taken to avoid touching the tip of the eye dropper to the lids, lashes, eye, or any surface outside the medicine bottle. To keep the medication in contact with the eye and to lessen the possibility of systemic side effects from medications entering the lacrimal drainage system, manual punctal occlusion may be performed. (After the drop is instilled, the patient is instructed to apply pressure to the medial canthus with the forefingers to seal the puncta).

Ointments are instilled by placing approximately a one-half inch ribbon of ointment from the tube into the lower lid pocket from one canthus to the other. Again, the tip of the tube should not be allowed to touch anything. This will help avoid contamination by organisms that could be transmitted to the other eye or to the next patient.

What the Patient Needs to Know

- Do not use medications more often or for longer periods than prescribed.

- Wash your hands before instilling medications.

- Do not touch the medication dropper or tube tip to the eye, eyelid, or any other surface.

- Report any medication side effects (red eye, discharge, pain) or worsening symptoms.

- Bring your medications to the next visit.

Chapter 2

Visual Acuity

KEY POINTS

- Visual acuity is tested at every visit.

- Visual acuity is usually tested with the patient wearing his or her current correction.

- Show the patient whole lines of letters, not isolated letters.

- Testing young children requires patience and kindness.

- Do not confront the suspected malingerer; he or she will not cooperate for vision testing.

OptP

Visual acuity is a primary indication of the health of the eye and visual system and is one of the first tests performed at the office visit. It is routinely checked at every visit. *Visual acuity* is defined as the smallest object resolvable by the eye at a given distance. It is expressed as a fraction in which the numerator denotes object size and the denominator denotes viewing distance in feet or meters. Visual acuity can be reduced by refractive error, ocular disease or injury, and/or neurologic disease.

The Visual Angle

OphA

CL

Optn

Testing visual acuity is a simple procedure based on fairly complex optical principles. The test demonstrates how well an eye distinguishes the size and shape of objects in the visual axis. The normal visual axis is composed of clear media (cornea, aqueous, lens, and vitreous) that focus light rays on the retinal fovea. Images that fall on the fovea and peripheral retina are then processed by the nervous system to produce the sense we know as vision.

The *visual angle* is defined as the angle that an object's outermost rays subtend on the retina and is measured in degrees or minutes of arc (Figure 2-1). At a given distance, a larger object subtends a larger angle; the same object subtends a larger angle when it is closer to the eye. The details of an object are what make it identifiable. For instance, an "E" and an "H" would look the same if the details within the outermost boundaries were not resolvable by the eye. An eye can resolve the details of an object when it can distinguish spatially separated parts of that object. The minimum angle resolvable by the normal human eye is about 1 minutes (min) of arc.

The symbols or *optotypes*—letters, numbers, pictures, etc—used on standard visual acuity charts are constructed so that each section of the symbol subtends 1 min of arc, and the whole symbol subtends 5 min of arc (Figure 2-2). The standard testing distance is 20 feet (ft) (6 meters [m]) for distance or 14 inches (in) for near. Because the testing distance is fixed, the size of the objects on the chart are varied to reflect different levels of visual ability. The size is expressed as the reciprocal of the distance at which the letter subtends 5 min of arc (eg, the 20/400 letter subtends 5 min of arc at 400 ft) and is written as the denominator. The numerator is the actual test distance, 20 ft. Another way to understand this fraction is to say that the denominator is the distance at which a viewer with normal vision can identify the same letter. For example, a normally sighted person can read the 20/60 size letters at 60 ft while the 20/60 level viewer can distinguish them from no farther than the 20-ft testing distance.

The Vision Chart

OptA

OphA

CL

Optn

The Snellen visual acuity chart is used most often in the clinical setting and is made up of certain letters of our alphabet. However, there are instances when other types of objects must be used because the patient is too young, not literate, not familiar with our alphabet, etc. Other charts employ simple, easily recognizable drawings or the letters E or C printed in different orientations (Figure 2-3). The patient is asked to identify the direction of the open end of the E or the break in the C. If the patient cannot or is reluctant to speak (eg, non-English speaking or young child), the patient can match pictures or use hand signals to identify the individual optotypes.

The charts themselves may be affixed to the wall opposite the examining chair, suspended in front of a light box, or projected onto the far wall via a system of mirrors. The latter method eliminates the need for a room that is 20 ft long and, therefore, maximizes office space. The

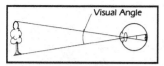

Figure 2-1. The visual angle is the angle of the outermost rays of an object subtended at the eye. (Drawing by Edmund Pett.) (Reprinted from Herrin MP. *Ophthalmic Examination and Basic Skills*. Thorofare, NJ: SLACK Incorporated; 1990.)

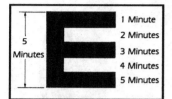

Figure 2-2. An E subtends an angle of 5 min of arc. (Drawing by Edmund Pett.) (Reprinted from Herrin MP. *Ophthalmic Examination and Basic Skills*. Thorofare, NJ: SLACK Incorporated; 1990.)

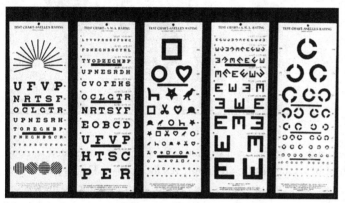

Figure 2-3. Charts A and B: Snellen letters; chart C: pictures and geometric shapes; chart D: tumbling E; and chart E: Landolt rings. (Reprinted from Herrin MP. *Ophthalmic Examination and Basic Skills*. Thorofare, NJ: SLACK Incorporated; 1990.)

optotypes are printed on a glass slide that is either inserted or permanently installed into a projector so that the chart appears on a mirror and/or silver screen for viewing. Standard bulbs provide background illumination, and each projector has manufacturer's instructions for setting up the instrument at the proper distance.

Testing Strategy

Distant Vision

Evaluating visual acuity is usually the first test performed at each office visit. (If the patient requires urgent treatment or if fusional status is in question, visual acuity may be tested later in the exam). The patient is seated comfortably in the exam chair, resting against the chair back. By convention, the right eye is tested first, so the left eye is occluded with an opaque paddle or mask. If the patient uses his or her hand (not recommended) to occlude the nontested eye, care must be taken that there is no view through the fingers (Figure 2-4) or that there is no pressure applied to the globe. Such pressure can temporarily change the refractive error and raise the intraocular pressure. Ordinarily, if the patient is wearing spectacles or contact lenses with a current prescription, vision is tested while the patient is wearing them. The patient should look through the top, distance portion of a multifocal spectacle lenses. If the patient's previous visual acuity is known, it will save some time to start the test with a line of letters 1 or 2 levels larger; it is not necessary to begin every test with the 20/400 E.

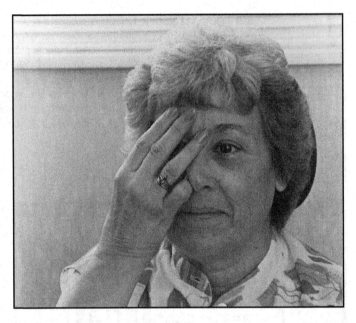

Figure 2-4. The patient can peek through his or her fingers if the hand is used as an occluder. (Photo by Mark Arrigoni.) (Reprinted from Herrin MP. *Ophthalmic Examination and Basic Skills*. Thorofare, NJ: SLACK Incorporated; 1990.)

This test is usually performed in dim illumination so that the pupil is not stimulated to constrict (which increases the depth of focus and artificially improves the acuity). This is part of the standardization of the test. Under certain circumstances (eg, an eye with a cataract), the vision may be tested in bright light as well to demonstrate that light actually diminishes vision and treatment is required.

If the patient is not familiar with the testing procedure, he or she may be shown a section of the chart with several lines visible and asked, "Can you make out any letters on the chart?" If the patient answers "Yes," then he or she may be asked to read the smallest line easily readable. The patient should be encouraged to read whole lines in order from left to right. If only 1 or 2 letters on a line are missed, the patient should then be asked to try to read the letters on the next smallest line. He or she will probably be able to correctly identify 1 or 2 letters on this line. Visual acuity is then recorded as the smallest line on which the patient correctly identified more than half the letters minus the number of letters missed (eg, VA = 20/40 -1) plus any correct letters from the next line (eg, VA = 20/40 -1/+2). Once the patient has read the smallest line possible, visual acuity for each eye is recorded.

It is always preferable to have a patient view a whole line of letters rather than single optotypes because distinguishing between letters is as important as distinguishing parts of a letter. This is especially significant when testing children because those with amblyopia are better able to identify single letters and the end letters of a line than letters bound on 2 sides by other letters. This is called the *crowding phenomenon*. Mild amblyopia may be missed if the child is presented with solitary objects to identify. Also, if an amblyopic child is being treated, follow-up testing with single optotypes may give a false impression of the eye's progress.

If the vision in either eye with proper correction is not 20/20, using a pinhole to try to improve vision will indicate whether or not there is a problem with the media (cornea or lens). A pinhole paddle is attached to the occluder mask (Figure 2-5) and contains multiple pinholes. Each 1.5- to 2-mm pinhole limits the light rays entering the eye to only the parallel rays, which do not have to be refracted to be focused on the macula. If the vision improves with the use of a pinhole,

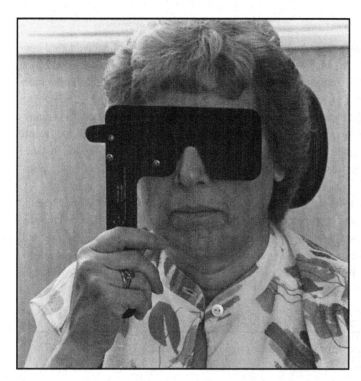

Figure 2-5. Some occluders have a pinhole attached that can be flipped into place. (Photo by Mark Arrigoni.) (Reprinted from Herrin MP. *Ophthalmic Examination and Basic Skills.* Thorofare, NJ: SLACK Incorporated; 1990.)

there may be some amount of uncorrected refractive error present. With the proper correction, the vision is usually improvable to at least the level found with the pinhole. If the pinhole does not improve the patient's acuity, then some nonrefractive problem, such as macular degeneration, may be responsible for the decreased vision.

Sometimes, a patient cannot discern even the 20/400 letter with the best correction in place. If feasible, the patient should be walked toward a wall chart until he or she can just distinguish the letter. Recalling that the numerator represents the testing distance, the vision would be recorded as 3/400 if that distance was 3 ft from the chart.

If the patient is not easily movable, the assistant can test the vision by holding up 1 to 4 fingers at different distances from the patient. This is recorded as *count fingers* (CF) at the farthest distance at which a correct count is obtained. For example, if the patient can correctly count the number of fingers held up at 3 ft but not at 4 ft, it is recorded as CF at 3 ft.

If the patient cannot count fingers at any distance, the assistant can try waving his or her hand back and forth at different distances from the patient. It is easier for the eye to see an object in motion, so this test differs from the count fingers strategy with regard to both the size of the target (whole hand) and its motion. Vision at this level is recorded as *hand motion* (eg, HM at 2 ft).

When vision is severely reduced, the patient may only be able to see the difference between light and dark. If the patient can accurately identify when a light is being shown to the eye, it is recorded as *light perception* (LP); if the patient can detect the *direction* from which the light is being shone, this is recorded as *light perception with projection* (LP c̄ P). When a patient cannot see this light or even the most powerful light (eg, the maximum setting on the indirect ophthalmoscope), this represents total blindness and is recorded as *no light perception* (NLP).

Near Vision

Near vision is measured at a standard distance of 14 in, and the "chart" is a handheld card containing lines of numbers or text. Again, vision in each eye is tested separately, and any correction for near is used (ie, the bifocal segment or reading glasses). This test is done in bright illumination. Near vision may be recorded in 1 of 3 standard notations. The Jaeger system (J1, J2, J3, etc) is a century-old standard in which the lower numerals represent better vision. For instance, J3 is equivalent to 20/40, and J1+ is 20/20. Another notation is the point system used commercially to denote print size, with N3 being 20/20 and higher numbers indicating poorer vision. Finally, the distance equivalent, a recalibration for the near test, can be used (20/20, 20/50, etc); these are usually printed on the near card.

When young or illiterate patients are being tested, pictures or a rotating letter (E or C) can be used. With very young children, the examiner can present uniform small objects and record the size of the object that the child can see well enough to pick up (eg, "picks up 3 mm object"). Small, round candies make an attractive target that also rewards the child, but the assistant should ask for the parents' permission before giving these to a child, and care must be taken that they will not be injurious to the child.

What the Patient Needs to Know

- Your vision is checked with your glasses on. (Let the assistant know if these are someone else's glasses!)

- If you use your hand to cover your eye, use the palm and do not press on the eyeball.

- Read all the letters on a line in order from left to right, even if you have to guess at some.

- When reading the near card, use your bifocal segment or reading glasses.

Factitious Visual Loss

Sometimes patients falsely claim visual loss in one or both eyes. There are 2 categories of factitious visual loss: *malingering* and *hysterical*. The malingering patient deliberately feigns visual loss for some kind of personal or financial gain, such as monetary compensation or to get attention. Hysterical visual loss usually results from emotional distress, such as witnessing a tragedy or experiencing a wrenching life change. Hysterical patients claim bilateral visual loss and differ from malingerers in that they truly believe they are blind; this may represent a psychological escape from their environment and often results in complete dependence.

With either type of false visual loss, uncovering and documenting it will call for some creative testing strategies. It is very helpful if the assistant has a high index of suspicion before the patient enters the room (eg, worker's compensation, litigation) or before the actual exam begins. It is important that the patient not be confronted with this suspicion of faking because this may affect the success of the testing. Also, the accusation may be false.

Before the patient enters the room, isolate the smallest line on the Snellen chart (20/10, if possible). If the patient is claiming visual loss in only one eye, it will be easier to discover if the loss is real. The "bad" eye should be tested first on the isolated small line, with the assistant encouraging guessing and persuading the patient to read successively larger lines. If the patient thought the original line was 20/20, he or she may tire of being pushed by the time the 20/30 or 20/40 line is presented and start "guessing" correctly. This gives a baseline from which to cajole even better vision from the patient.

The good vision in one normal eye can be used to elicit the true vision in the "bad" eye. There are several tests that can be used to prove good vision in both eyes when the patient is falsely claiming poor vision in one eye. Each of these tests depends on the patient's not knowing which eye is being used or that the test requires good vision in both eyes. Accordingly, these tests are performed with both eyes open.

Stereoacuity is a test of fine binocular visual function that uses polarizing glasses, enabling each eye to see something different from the other (see Chapter 11). The test booklet has progressively more difficult 3-dimensional pictures. The patient who correctly identifies most or all of these test items has proven good vision in both eyes.

Another test that uses polarizing glasses is the Polaroid vectograph—a distance test using Snellen letters. On any given line, each eye sees different letters. Therefore, if the patient reads the whole line, both eyes are seeing equally well.

The Worth 4 Dot test also uses glasses that separate what the 2 eyes see. A red lens allows the eye behind it to see only the red lights of the flashlight, and a green lens allows only the green lights to be seen. If the patient identifies all the lights, then both eyes are seeing; however, actual acuity is not determinable by this test. It is most useful if the patient is claiming *no* vision in an eye. In order to discover what each eye sees, the examiner must be sure that the patient keeps both eyes open. Using only one eye, the patient can easily continue to feign monocular visual loss.

There are objective tests of monocular visual loss that can also indicate the real level of vision. The optokinetic nystagmus (OKN) drum or strip can be used to establish the existence of vision, and the size of the stripes or figures on the drum will indicate the level of vision. Just as the eyes have a normal nystagmus while a person is riding in a vehicle and watching telephone poles go by, the OKN movement is a normal response to the drum movement. The examiner turns the drum slowly in front of the patient's eyes; the seeing eye automatically follows the stripes on the drum. While the patient is watching the turning drum, the assistant alternately covers the patient's eyes. If one eye truly cannot see, then it will stop moving.

Another objective test is to have the patient slowly read a small line of numbers on a near card with both eyes open and alternately introduce a 4 diopter prism base-out in front of each eye. While watching the patient's eyes, the examiner will notice that the eye behind the prism shifts *in* to fuse with the other eye. If both eyes do this, it indicates that both eyes see the small numbers equally well.

A few other tests and observations may prove useful. When a patient claims visual loss in both eyes, it is important and helpful to observe his or her behavior. Someone who is severely visually impaired will not come to the office alone. The assistant may be able to demonstrate tunnel visual fields by performing a confrontation test (see Chapter 5) at different distances and observing the extent of the borders. The field should be larger at a greater distance. Finally, electrophysiologic testing can be done to evaluate the status of the visual system and to compare the function between the 2 eyes.

Chapter 3

Lensometry, Transposition, and Geneva Lens Measure

KEY POINTS

- Focus the lensometer eyepiece before measuring a lens, being careful not to over minus.

- Make sure the frames rest evenly on the stage.

- Trifocal power is usually half the bifocal power.

- If the mires cannot be centered, there is ground-in prism.

- Do not scratch a plastic lens when marking the optical center (OC) or measuring with lens clock.

The Lensometer

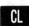

One of the most important tasks performed by the assistant in the office is assessing the power of the spectacle correction worn by the patient. This measurement is made on either a manual or automated instrument called a *lensmeter* (commonly called a *lensometer* in the United States). The patient's spectacle correction should be recorded at the initial visit and at any time a new prescription has been filled. In addition to measuring the power, the lensometer is used to measure the added power of a bifocal or trifocal segment or any prism ground into the lens. The instrument can be used to locate the ocular centers (OCs) of the lenses, which are then compared to the visual axes and evaluated for intentionally or unintentionally induced prism. Whenever a patient is not comfortable with a new prescription, the power, prism, OCs, and base curves must be evaluated for each lens.

Instrumentation

The lensometer is a tabletop instrument used to neutralize spectacle lenses. It consists of an ocular for viewing the measurement images (mires), a flat stage or table for supporting the spectacle frame, a power dial, and an axis dial (Figure 3-1).

Adjusting the Eyepiece

As with any instrument with a reticle (also called an *ocular* or *eyepiece*), the lensometer must be focused for the examiner's eye. Because the reticle does not correct for astigmatism, the examiner should wear his or her own glasses if they contain a significant astigmatic correction. The reticle adjustment is critical for obtaining an accurate measurement.

With the power dial set at zero, a piece of white paper is placed where the spectacle lens will be positioned (Figure 3-2). Against this background, the cross hairs in the reticle are focused by first turning the reticle fully counterclockwise and then rotating it slowly clockwise until the cross hairs first appear to be in focus. The counterclockwise rotation puts a plus lens in front of the examiner's eye; rotating the reticle back only as far as the earliest focus helps to avoid overminusing the examiner's eye and introducing error to the spectacle lens measurement. The eye naturally accommodates on the reticle because it is perceived to be near, so a reticle set a little to the left of zero (a minus lens) will not be a problem.

Performing Lensometry

The spectacles are placed on the stage so the temple pieces point backward and both lenses are supported evenly on the stage. The upper distance portion of the right lens is centered against the lens post, and the lens holder is carefully positioned against the front of the lens (Figure 3-3).

One of 2 types of targets (mires) will be visible through the eyepiece: crossed linear mires (spaced differently) or dots (circular formation). The center of the mires must be centered in the eyepiece. The spectacles can be moved horizontally on the stage, and/or the stage can be moved vertically to center the mires.

Because instruments with linear mires are more often used, the method for lens measurement will be demonstrated with these. The lines in one direction of the cross are thinner and lie very close together, while the lines in the other direction are thicker and more widely spaced (Figure 3-4). The assistant turns the power dial on the right side of the instrument to focus the mires. If

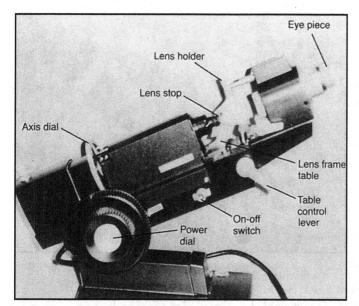

Figure 3-1. Example of a manual lensometer. (Reprinted with permission from Reichert Ophthalmic Instruments.)

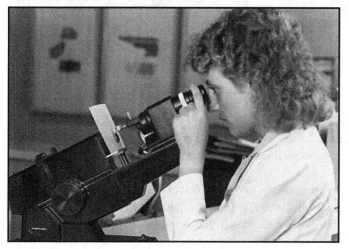

Figure 3-2. A white piece of paper provides an excellent background for eyepiece adjustment. (Photo by Mark Arrigoni.) (Reprinted from Herrin MP. *Ophthalmic Examination and Basic Skills*. Thorofare, NJ: SLACK Incorporated; 1990.)

all the lines are focused simultaneously, the lens is spherical (ie, there is no cylinder power). Zero on the power dial represents plano; the numbers above zero are plus sphere, and the numbers below zero (sometimes printed in red) are minus sphere. The spherical power of the lens is read directly from the dial when the mires are in focus.

If all the mires cannot be focused at the same time, then the lens contains some cylindrical correction. In this case, the sphere is determined first. If the reading is to be in plus cylinder notation, then the thin lines must be focused first and by the least plus position of the power dial (Figure 3-5). The axis wheel on top of the rear of the instrument is turned so that the mires are straight. If the thick mires are in focus at the least plus position on the power dial, then the axis wheel must be turned 90 degrees. This changes the relationship of the 2 focus positions so that the thin mires are now focused at less plus (or more minus) than the thick mires. The least plus reading is recorded as the spherical portion of the lens. The thick mires are then focused by turning the power dial in the plus direction. The second focus position on the power dial is noted, and

Figure 3-3. Gently place the lens in the holder so as not to scratch the plastic lenses. (Photo by Mark Arrigoni.) (Reprinted from Herrin MP. *Ophthalmic Examination and Basic Skills*. Thorofare, NJ: SLACK Incorporated; 1990.)

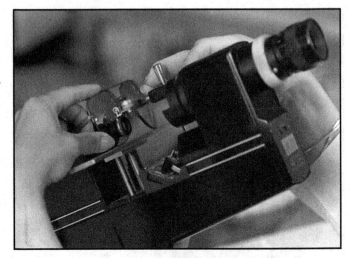

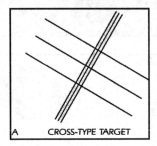

Figure 3-4. Common lensometer mires. (Reprinted from Herrin MP. *Ophthalmic Examination and Basic Skills*. Thorofare, NJ: SLACK Incorporated; 1990.)

the algebraic difference between the 2 focus positions is recorded as the plus cylinder. (It may help to think of the power dial as a number line.) The number indicated on the axis wheel is the axis of the cylinder.

Minus cylinder is easily read by focusing the thin mires first at the most plus power dial position, adjusting the axis wheel to accomplish this. The minus cylinder is then determined by finding the difference in the 2 focus positions as the power dial is moved in the minus direction to focus the thick mires.

Example 1.   The thin mires are clear at -2.00 on the dial:
-2.00 sphere
The thick mires are clear at +1.00 on the dial:
-2.00 to +1.00 is +3.00 cylinder
The axis where all mires are straight is 95.
The lens power is -2.00 + 3.00 x 95.

Example 2.   The thin mires are clear at -2.00:
-2.00 sphere
The thick mires are clear at -5.00:
-2.00 to -5.00 is -3.00 cylinder
The axis setting is 135.
The lens power is -2.00 - 3.00 x 135.

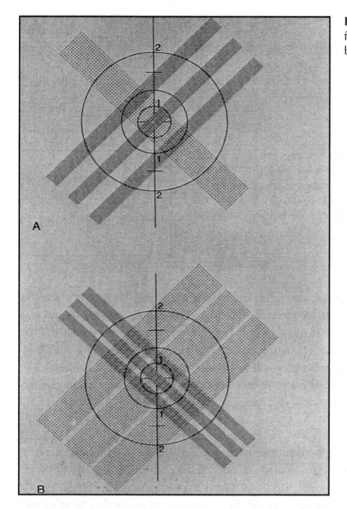

Measuring a Multifocal Lens

The bifocal or trifocal segment of a lens is an extra plus spherical lens for near vision that is ground onto the distance lens. The amount of power in this extra lens is a calculation of the difference between its measured power and the spherical portion of the distance lens. The power dial is set at the focus of the distance sphere (thin mires), or this number is remembered. The stage is then moved up so that the mires of the bifocal or trifocal segment are centered in the reticle. The power dial is then rotated to refocus the thin mires. The new power will always be more plus than the distance sphere, and the number recorded is the difference between the new power and the distance sphere. It is recorded as an *add* to the lens and is usually +1.00 to +3.00 diopters (D).

For example, suppose the distance portion of the lens reads -2.50 + 1.00 x 085. After sliding the stage up to measure the bifocal segment and adjusting the power dial, the thin mires are now clear at -0.25. The add is +2.25, the difference between -2.50 and -0.25. The prescription for this bifocal lens is written:

-2.50 + 1.00 x 085   +2.25 add

The trifocal segment is placed above the near bifocal segment and is for intermediate distance. Also, it will be more plus than the distance sphere but not as much as the bifocal. Usually

Figure 3-6. A plus lens is 2 prisms base to base, and a minus lens is 2 prisms apex to apex. (Reprinted from Herrin MP. *Ophthalmic Examination and Basic Skills.* Thorofare, NJ: SLACK Incorporated; 1990.)

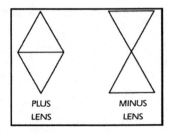

Figure 3-7. Base-in prism is induced when the optical center separation is greater than the interpupillary distance (IPD). Base-out prism is induced when the OC separation is less than the IPD. (Drawing by Edmund Pett.) (Reprinted from Herrin MP. *Ophthalmic Examination and Basic Skills.* Thorofare, NJ: SLACK Incorporated; 1990.)

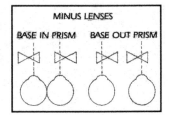

the trifocal segment is half the extra power of the bifocal, but sometimes the patient's specific visual requirements at an intermediate distance (eg, reading sheet music, performing tasks at arm's length) warrant special attention to this segment. These powers are typically up to +1.50 D.

Patients in some professions, such as plumbers or electricians, have visual requirements in upgaze rather than downgaze. Their spectacles will be constructed with the bifocal/trifocal segments at the top of the distance lens. These segments are measured in the same manner as the more usual segments found at the bottom of the lens.

Locating the Optical Centers

A plus lens is produced by putting 2 prisms base to base; a minus lens is 2 prisms apex to apex (Figure 3-6). The optical center (OC) of a lens is where the 2 prisms meet and is represented by the center of the crossed mires in the lensometer. Most lensometers have a row of inked pins that can be used to mark the OC of each lens. The distance between the 2 OCs is compared to the patient's interpupillary distance (IPD), or the OC of each lens is checked for proper alignment with the eye's visual axis. If one or both OCs do not align with the visual axis, the patient may experience asthenopic symptoms, such as blurring, a pulling sensation, or eyestrain. These symptoms may be due to the prism induced when wearing the spectacles.

The amount of induced prism and the direction of the prism are determined by both the prescription and the position of the eyes. If the prescription has a spherical equivalent of minus and the OC is displaced toward the nose, then the eye is looking through base-out prism; if the OC is displaced toward the ear, the eye is looking through base-in prism (Figure 3-7). With a plus lens, because the bases of the prisms form the OC, the opposite is true (eg, the OC displaced nasally produces base-in prism) (Figure 3-8). Vertical prism may be induced when the OCs are displaced upward or downward.

Although unintentional induced prism can cause eyestrain, sometimes prism is deliberately induced in the spectacles of patients who have a symptomatic extraocular muscle imbalance. The formula for calculating the amount of induced prism is as follows: OC displacement (in cm) x lens power = amount of prism. (Lens power is spherical equivalent or the power in the meridian of the displacement.)

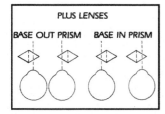

PLUS LENSES

BASE OUT PRISM   BASE IN PRISM

Figure 3-8. Base-out prism is induced when the OC separation is greater than the IPD. Base-in prism is induced when the OC separation is less than the IPD. (Drawing by Edmund Pett.) (Reprinted from Herrin MP. *Ophthalmic Examination and Basic Skills.* Thorofare, NJ: SLACK Incorporated; 1990.)

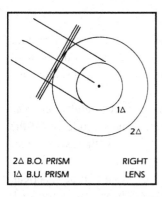

2△ B.O. PRISM   RIGHT
1△ B.U. PRISM   LENS

Figure 3-9. The amount of prism and its direction are determined by the position of the target on the rings. (Reprinted from Herrin MP. *Ophthalmic Examination and Basic Skills.* Thorofare, NJ: SLACK Incorporated; 1990.)

Measuring Ground-In Prism

When the mires cannot be centered in the lensometer, the prism has been ground into the spectacle lens.

The reticle contains concentric circles that can be used to measure small amounts of prism. There may also be a dial at the opposite end of the reticle carrier that measures higher amounts of prism. The amount of prism is read from the dial or from the nearest ring to which the center of the mires can be moved. The direction of the prism is determined by where the mires are located relative to the reticle center. For instance, if the right lens is being read and the mires' center falls to the left and above the reticle center, then the prism is base-out and base-up (Figure 3-9).

Transposition

Whether the lens power is recorded in plus or minus cylinder, it is possible to convert from one to the other with an algebraic transposition. There are 3 steps in the transposition:

1. The cylinder power is added to the sphere, paying attention to the sign of the cylinder.
2. The sign of the cylinder is changed.
3. The axis is changed by 90 degrees.

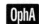

OptA

OphA

Optn

Example 1.	-2.00 + 3.00 x 075 =
transposition:	1. -2.00 + 3.00 = +1.00 sph
	2. change cylinder sign = -3.00 cyl
	3. 75 + 90 degrees = 165 axis
result:	+1.00 - 3.00 x 165

Example 2.   +3.00 - 1.00 x 090
transposition: 1. +3.00 + (-1.00) = +2.00 sph
                  2. change cylinder sign = +1.00 cyl
                  3. 90 + 90 degrees = 180 axis
result: +2.00 + 1.00 x 180

Geneva Lens Clock

The Geneva lens clock (or lens measure) is a handheld instrument that measures the surface power of a spectacle lens in diopters. It has a round gauge on front and 3 pins on the bottom. When the pins contact a flat surface and the clock itself is held perpendicular to that surface, the gauge should read zero.

The middle pin of the clock is placed on the OC of the lens. The clock is carefully held perpendicular to the lens. The clock is rotated on the lens using the center pin as a fulcrum. If the gauge reading does not change during rotation, then the lens is spherical. If the reading does change, then the lens is toric (ie, has cylinder).

Cylinder is usually ground onto the back surface of a lens; thus, the front will be spherical. To read lens power with the lens clock, first measure the front surface. Then measure the back surface, turning the clock to look for cylinder. If no cylinder is present, the lens power is found by algebraically adding the 2 powers. For example, if the front surface is +10.00 sph and the back surface is -7.00 sph, then +10.00 + (-7.00) = +3.00 sph (Figure 3-10.)

If there is cylinder on the back surface of the lens, first determine the highest and lowest readings by observing the dial as you turn the clock. Also, note the approximate axis where the highest and lowest readings occur. The amount of cylinder present is the difference between the highest and lowest reading, as on a lensometer. To read the lens in minus cylinder using the lens measure, use the *weakest* of the 2 back surface readings; you will also use its axis as the axis for the lens power. Suppose the front surface read +5.00 sph, and the back surface read -4.00 at 30 degrees and -7.00 at 120 degrees. There are -3.00 D of cylinder present on the back curve [-7.00 - (-4.00)]. Using the weaker curve, we have +5.00 + (-4.00) = +1.00. The prescription is thus +1.00 - 3.00 x 030 (Figure 3-11).

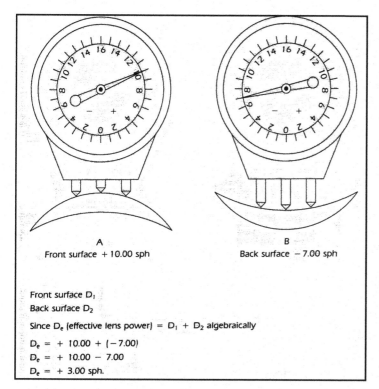

Figure 3-10. Geneva lens measure spherical reading. (Reprinted from Blair B, Appleton B, Garber N, Crowe M, Alven MT. *Opticianry, Ocularistry and Ophthalmic Technology.* Thorofare, NJ: SLACK Incorporated; 1990.)

A
Front surface + 10.00 sph

B
Back surface − 7.00 sph

Front surface D_1

Back surface D_2

Since D_e (effective lens power) = D_1 + D_2 algebraically

D_e = + 10.00 + (− 7.00)

D_e = + 10.00 − 7.00

D_e = + 3.00 sph.

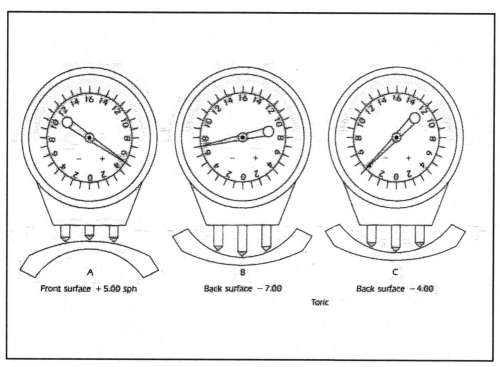

A
Front surface + 5.00 sph

B
Back surface − 7.00

C
Back surface − 4.00

Toric

Figure 3-11. Geneva lens measure, cylindrical reading. (Reprinted from Blair B, Appleton B, Garber N, Crowe M, Alven MT. *Opticianry, Ocularistry and Ophthalmic Technology.* Thorofare, NJ: SLACK Incorporated; 1990.)

Chapter 4

Keratometry

KEY POINTS

- Focus the eyepiece before beginning the measurement.

- Let the patient blink normally to keep the cornea smooth.

- Make sure the patient is comfortable while positioned at the instrument.

- Loosely lock the instrument to avoid accidentally misaligning it during the measurement.

- Keep the mires centered and focused at all times.

- Use the crosses both horizontally and vertically for the most accurate measurement.

Instrumentation

The cornea is a powerful refracting surface, providing two-thirds of approximately 60 D of the eye's total refracting power. The keratometer is an instrument that measures the front curvature of the cornea, providing measurements in both millimeters of radius of curvature and diopters of optical power. The dioptric power is used to estimate the amount of corneal astigmatism for visual correction or for calculating the power of an intraocular replacement lens after cataract surgery. The radius of curvature measurement is useful when fitting contact lenses because their base curves (which rest against the cornea) are specified in millimeters.

The keratometer rests on a tabletop or is attached to an arm of the chairside stand. It consists of an eyepiece for the examiner, a chin rest for the patient, knobs to adjust the height of the instrument or the patient's chin, a focusing knob, and dials for aligning the target circles (mires) (Figure 4-1).

An illuminated circle at the front of the instrument is reflected on the cornea. The circular mires of this particular instrument have a cross at each side and a dash above and below. The keratometer splits this image into 3 identical circles in a reverse "L" configuration (Figure 4-2), and the measurement is taken by moving the circles relative to each other with the instrument dials. The mires will be large and round if the cornea is flat and spherical. Smaller mires indicate a steeper cornea; oval mires indicate the presence of astigmatism.

Measuring Corneal Curvature

With the keratometer turned on, the eyepiece is adjusted to focus the cross hairs for the examiner's eye in the same manner as for the lensometer (see Chapter 3). The patient should be seated comfortably in the examining chair, and the keratometer should be brought toward the patient's face. The patient places his or her chin in the chin rest and rests his or her head against the forehead bar or band. If necessary, the patient's head can be repositioned using the chin rest elevator and/or adjuster. The assistant should make sure the patient is comfortable before beginning the measurement. The patient should be instructed to look at the target in the instrument, at the center of the circle, or at the reflection of his or her own eye at all times. If the patient's vision is extremely poor, or if he or she doesn't seem to understand where to look, a penlight can be shown through the eyepiece. (This should not be done during the reading, but it will give the patient an idea of where to fixate.) The patient should also be reminded to blink normally throughout the test because this helps keep the corneal surface smooth. A drop of artificial tears may be needed if the cornea is dry, but the eyes should be gently blotted before taking the reading.

The barrel of the keratometer is directed at the right eye, and its height is adjusted so the lighted circle reflects onto the patient's cornea. This may be difficult for the examiner to see, but the light from a penlight shown through the eyepiece can be easily centered on the cornea to grossly align the instrument. The examiner, looking through the eyepiece, should be able to see the 3 mires. If they are blurred or doubled, the focusing knob or joystick is used to move the barrel forward or back until the 3 circles are single and in sharp focus. Finer adjustments of the barrel position should place the cross hairs in the center of the lower right circle. If the 3 circles are not completely separated from each other, the horizontal dial on the left and vertical dial on the right are turned to move the circles apart. Once it is properly aligned, the barrel should be locked

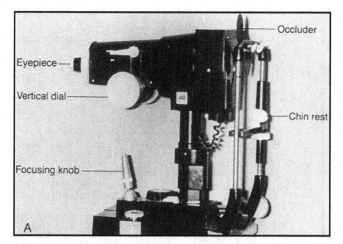

Figure 4-1. Two types of commonly used manual keratometers. (Reprinted with permission from Reichert Ophthalmic Instruments.)

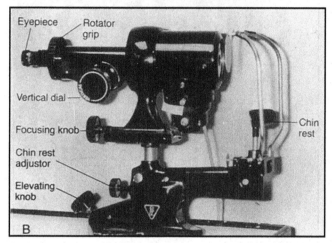

What the Patient Needs to Know

- Keep your head firmly in position for the test.

- Look at the target or at your own eye's reflection to maintain eye position.

- Keep both eyes open.

- Remember to blink normally.

in place with the lock screw on the left. Do not lock it too tightly because the alignment may need fine adjustment during the measurement.

To begin the measurement, the keratometer barrel is rotated either clockwise or counterclockwise to align the crosses of the 2 lower circles so that they are exactly opposite each other. The left horizontal dial is then turned so that the crosses are moved toward each other until they are superimposed on each other and appear to be a single cross connecting the 2 circles.

Next, the right vertical dial is turned to superimpose the dashes between the upper and lower circles on the right so that it appears to be a single dash. During both of these maneuvers, the mires must be kept centered on the patient's cornea and sharply focused.

Figure 4-2. Lensometer mires. Unaligned horizontal plus signs (top) are aligned (bottom) using the axis dial. (Reprinted with permission from WB Saunders.)

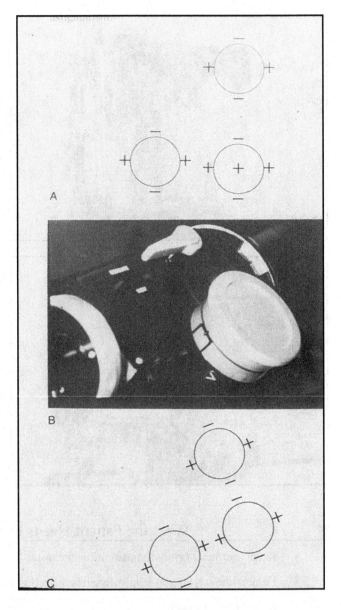

Once the crosses and dashes have been superimposed, the measurements can be read directly from the instrument. The numbers indicated on the horizontal and vertical dials are recorded in diopters, and the 2 axes corresponding to the 2 dioptric powers may be read from the axis dial. By convention, the lower number, corresponding to the flattest corneal meridian, and its axis are written first.

Example: OD 42.25 x 175 / 43.50 x 85

There is a shorthand version of this reading that leaves out the axis of the flatter meridian, making the assumption that the 2 readings will always be 90 degrees apart.

Example :   OD 42.25 / 43.50 x 85

The assistant should record the readings before the keratometer is moved to measure the other eye.

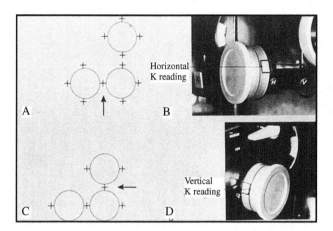

Figure 4-3. Use the plus signs for both horizontal and vertical readings to improve accuracy. (Reprinted from Cassin B, Hamed LM, eds. *Fundamentals for Ophthalmic Technical Personnel.* Philadelphia, Pa: WB Saunders Co; 1995.)

Measurement Problems

There are some caveats to be considered when using the keratometer. The instrument measures only the central 3 mm of the cornea and gives no information about the remaining 75% of the corneal surface. Also, because it depends on the reflection of light from a smooth surface, corneal epithelial irregularities, such as punctate keratopathy, may render the mires unable to be focused. In this situation, an estimate of the curvature may be made, but distortion of the mires should also be noted along with the recorded data. Corneal topography, using a more sophisticated and expensive instrument, gives a detailed analysis of a larger area of the cornea as well as multiple measurements of dioptric power.

Sometimes the crosses and dashes of the keratometer mires cannot be precisely superimposed simultaneously. This may mean that the corneal surface is irregular or that the principal meridians are not 90 degrees apart. To get a more accurate reading, once the horizontal reading is taken, the barrel can be rotated so that the crosses are now vertical (Figure 4-3). The dial is turned to vertically superimpose them, and the power reading is taken from this dial. When this method is used, both axes must be recorded with their corresponding powers.

If the cornea is very steep, the keratometer readings may exceed the numbers on the dial. In order to extend the range of measurement, a +1.25-D or a +2.25-D trial frame lens can be taped to the face of the keratometer in the center of the lighted circle and over the hole (1.25D extends the keratometer range about 8 diopters). A chart provided by the manufacturer is then used to determine the true dioptric curvature of the cornea from the new reading.

Finally, when the surface of the cornea has been altered (as when refractive surgery has been performed), the keratometer readings are no longer accurate. Because the readings are based on the index of refraction of the cornea and surgery has changed this, using the direct reading will lead to incorrect calculations for intraocular lens choice, for instance. A formula must be used to arrive at a more accurate estimation of the corneal power.

To ensure accuracy, the keratometer must be periodically calibrated and properly maintained. For a full description of the care of this instrument, please refer to the Series title *Ophthalmic Instrumentation.*

Chapter 5

Informal Visual Fields

KEY POINTS

- Informal visual fields are a screening test for visual system problems.

- Defects that respect the vertical or horizontal meridian should be further investigated with formal visual fields.

- Use your open eye opposite the eye being tested as the fixation point.

- Present the target midway between the patient and yourself.

- Record the visual field from the patient's point of view.

An integral part of the comprehensive eye exam is the evaluation of the extent and integrity of the visual field. A great deal of information can be gained by performing quick and easy informal field exams. These tests are done in the examining room and require no special equipment. The assistant who is familiar with the entire visual system will be able to get the most useful information from these tests. A complete discussion of this topic can be found in the Series title *Visual Fields*.

The Visual Field

The extent of the environment visible to the eye when it is fixated on an object is called the *visual field*. It extends about 60 degrees nasally and superiorly, about 70 degrees inferiorly, and about 90 degrees temporally (Figure 5-1). For the sake of evaluating defects in the visual field, it is divided into 4 quadrants: inferior, superior, left, and right. Defects in the normal, full visual field are caused by disease or injury in the visual system. Identifying visual field defects is a diagnostic tool used to localize the problem.

Light rays from an object in visual space travel in straight lines and are received by the retina *opposite* the location of the object. For example, light from an object in the right visual field hits the left side of the retina in each eye (ie, nasal retina of the right eye and temporal retina of the left eye). Light from an object below fixation (inferior visual field) hits superior retina in both eyes and so on. It is important to remember this relationship of the visual field to locations on the retina (spatial localization) when performing any type of visual field test.

The Visual System

The extent Light rays from the object of regard enter the eye and are refracted through clear media: the cornea, aqueous, lens, and vitreous. The light rays pass through the layers of the retina and stimulate the photoreceptor cells in the outer retina. Light is chemically transformed to electrical energy, which is then transmitted back through the retina to the ganglion cells of the inner retina. The nerve fibers (cell axons) from these cells exit the eye through the optic nerve. The millions of exiting nerve fibers come from the entire retina and are aligned in a particular pattern that divides the retina into inferior and superior sections (Figure 5-2). As the nerve fibers reach the posterior end of the optic nerves, they enter a structure called the *chiasm* (Figure 5-3). Here, the temporal fibers from each eye continue posteriorly on the same side of the brain (ipsilateral) while the nasal fibers cross to the other side of the brain (contralateral). This is how the brain is able to integrate the images from the 2 eyes into one. As the fibers exit the chiasm—right eye temporal fibers and left eye nasal fibers on the right, and right eye nasal fibers and left eye temporal fibers on the left—they travel through the right and left optic tracts to synapse at the lateral geniculate body. From there, the fibers spread out into the optic radiations and end in the occipital lobe, the most posterior part of the brain. Each section of the visual system has a specific type of visual field loss associated with it. The visual system is discussed in detail in the Series title *Ocular Anatomy and Physiology*.

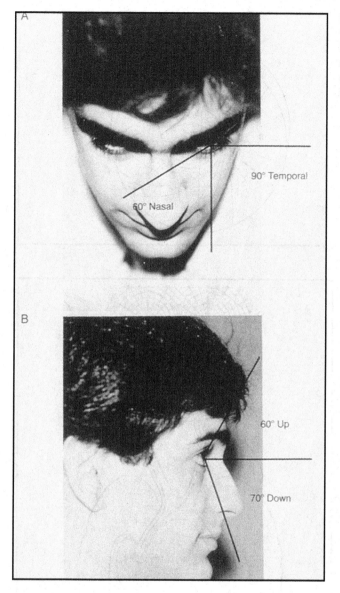

Figure 5-1. Normal extent of the visual field. (Reprinted from Cassin B, Hamed LM, eds. *Fundamentals for Ophthalmic Technical Personnel*. Philadelphia, Pa: WB Saunders Co; 1995.)

Pathology and the Visual Field

How does disease or injury in the visual system relate to changes in the visual field? An accurate visual field test has great diagnostic value because certain categories of visual field defects can localize a problem in the visual system that is not visible to the examiner.

Focal lesions of the retina, such as scars, have corresponding blind spots in opposite visual space. If a disease process, such as glaucoma or a retinal vascular occlusion, affects a section of the nerve fiber layer, then the visual field may show a defect that is either above or below the horizontal meridian but does not cross it (ie, respects the horizontal). A lesion at the chiasm, which lies over the pituitary gland, causes defects of the temporal side of the visual field in *both* eyes (bitemporal hemianopia). This is because the nasal nerve fibers from each eye cross at this point,

Figure 5-2. Diagram of the nerve fiber distribution in the right and left eyes. (A) Optic disc. (B) Radiating nasal fibers. (C) Vertical meridian that separates crossing nasal nerve fibers from the temporal uncrossed nerve fibers. (D) Horizontal raphe, which separates temporal superior retinal receptors from temporal inferior retinal receptors. (Reprinted from Garber N. *Visual Field Examination*. Thorofare, NJ: SLACK Incorporated; 1988.)

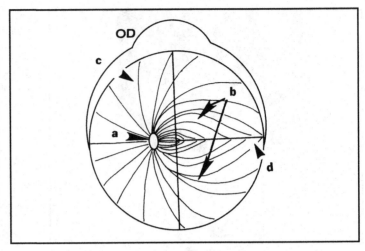

Figure 5-3. Visual system. Left nasal fibers (left visual space) cross at the chiasm to travel with right temporal fibers (left visual space) to the processing center in the posterior brain. (Reprinted from Cassin B, Hamed LM, eds. *Fundamentals for Ophthalmic Technical Personnel*. Philadelphia, Pa: WB Saunders Co; 1995.)

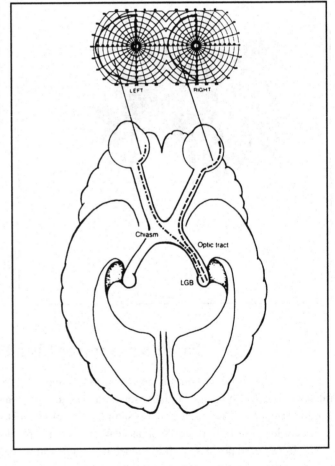

so both eyes can be affected by a single lesion. Posterior to the chiasm, the temporal fibers of one eye (nasal field) travel with the nasal fibers from the other eye (temporal field). A problem in this area will affect the *same side* of visual space in each eye's visual field (homonymous hemianopia). For example, a tumor in the right posterior brain may affect the right eye's temporal fibers (nasal or left visual space) and the left eye's nasal fibers (temporal or left visual space), which cross at the chiasm. Obviously, detailed formal visual field testing will be indicated for suspected serious visual system disorders. The suspicion of a problem, however, is often raised during routine informal visual field testing.

The Informal Visual Field

`OphT`

Informal visual field testing is done in the examining room and is considered a screening test. With it, the examiner can get a gross estimation of large visual field defects and their general locations. If such a defect is found, the patient will usually undergo formal testing with an instrument capable of detailing the defect under standardized conditions. There are 2 commonly used informal screening tests: the confrontation test and the Amsler grid. The confrontation test can detect and grossly define peripheral and/or large central defects, while the Amsler grid is a more sensitive test of the central visual field.

The Confrontation Visual Field Test

The assistant sits directly in front of the patient so that they are 2 or 3 ft apart (about an arm's length) and their eyes are on the same level. The patient is asked to cover his or her left eye with the palm of the hand, being sure not to apply pressure to the eye. The assistant then closes his or her right eye and instructs the patient to look only at the open eye at all times. In this way, the assistant's normal field of vision corresponds to the patient's and serves as the comparison for the test.

The assistant then presents 1 to 4 fingers in each of the 4 quadrants of the visual field and asks the patient to report the number of fingers being shown without looking directly at them. The fingers are presented midway between the patient and the assistant so each can see the targets equally well. The test is performed separately on each eye. This gross static test (ie, the fingers do not move once presented) can detect differences in the visual field from side to side (hemianopias) and above and below (altitudinal or arcuate).

If the patient cannot see the assistant's eye to maintain fixation, he or she may have a central blind spot (eg, macular degeneration). It is still important to determine if there is any other type of visual field defect that might be detected with peripheral testing. In this case, the patient can be asked to look at the assistant's face and to try to hold the eye steady while the fingers are presented peripheral to the central blind spot.

Kinetic visual field testing (a moving target) can establish gross peripheral boundaries, the size of large blind spots, or respect for the vertical or horizontal meridians. For this test, the assistant moves his or her fingers from the far periphery toward the center in each quadrant (Figure 5-4). Except for the inferotemporal quadrant, the fingers should not be immediately visible. The patient is instructed to report when the fingers first come into view. If the patient's visual field is normal, this point will be about the same time as the examiner sees the fingers.

There are some variations of the standard confrontation test that may be more sensitive for discovering hemianopias or altitudinal defects. One of these strategies involves presenting

Figure 5-4. The examiner presents a target (fingers) in the patient's right inferonasal field midway between them. (Reprinted from Herrin MP. *Ophthalmic Examination and Basic Skills.* Thorofare, NJ: SLACK Incorporated; 1990.)

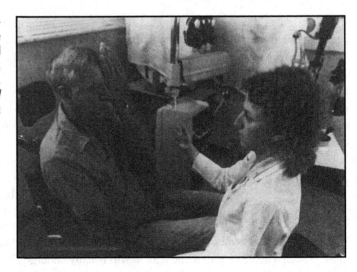

fingers in 2 quadrants at once and asking the patient to count the total number seen. If the targets are presented on either side of the vertical midline and the patient sees only the fingers on one side, this suggests hemianopic loss on the other side. Similarly, fingers seen only below the horizontal midline when they are presented both above and below suggests a superior altitudinal defect.

Another strategy for detecting differences in sensitivity is to use a brightly colored object, such as a red-topped eye drop bottle. The patient is asked if the color differs when the red top is shown on one side versus the other. Differences in actual color or brightness in one area of the visual field demonstrates loss of at least some of the normal perception of that color.

What the Patient Needs to Know

- Cover your eye completely without pressing on the eyeball.

- Maintain fixation on the assistant's open eye.

- Do not look in the direction of the assistant's hands.

- When the assistant's hands are moving toward you from the side, let the assistant know as soon as you see them.

 Testing With the Amsler Grid

Small blind spots in the central visual field will not be detected using the confrontation test because the target is too big. The Amsler grid is a near test designed to evaluate the central 20 degrees of the visual field (Figure 5-5). It consists of a 20 x 20 cm square made up of vertical and horizontal lines forming 5-mm squares. It may be printed black on a white background, or vice versa, and has a dot in the center for fixation.

The patient wears near correction, if needed. Testing each eye separately, the patient is instructed to focus only on the central dot of the grid and to report any distortion of lines, dark or blank spots, etc. This test is an excellent, fairly sensitive method of detecting early macular changes or of following the resolution of optic nerve disorders. The test can be sent home with the patient for regular self-evaluation.

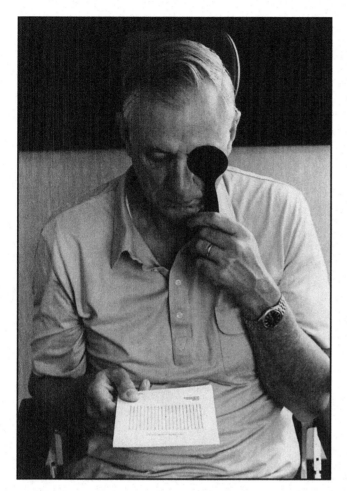

Figure 5-5. The patient views the central dot of the Amsler grid to localize any central defects in the visual field. (Reprinted from Herrin MP. *Ophthalmic Examination and Basic Skills.* Thorofare, NJ: SLACK Incorporated; 1990.)

What the Patient Needs to Know

- Use your bifocal or reading glasses for this test.

- Keep your eye focused on the central dot.

- Use this test at home to look for any changes in your central vision. Call the office immediately if you detect any change.

Chapter 6

The Pupil Evaluation

- Check pupils on every new patient and patients with recent visual loss.

- Check pupils before instilling any drops.

- Get verification of a questionable relative afferent pupillary defect (RAPD).

- Check pupils in dim illumination with a bright light.

- Move the light rapidly between the eyes when checking for a RAPD.

- The patient must be looking at a distant target for the pupil exam.

- Check the near reaction if the light reaction is abnormal.

- Unusual pupil function can also be observed with the slit lamp.

Normal function of the pupil is another indicator of the overall health of the entire visual system and is readily tested in the office setting. A pupil exam is performed on every new patient and on any patient with a new complaint of visual loss or eye pain. Assessment of pupil function should be done before any drops are instilled in the eye and before the cornea is touched (eg, applanation tension or Schirmer test).

OphA
RA

OptA

Anatomy and Innervation of the Pupil

The pupil is the central aperture in the iris and regulates the amount of light that enters the eye. Its size is governed by 2 opposing muscles: the dilator and the sphincter. The dilator muscle is radially aligned so that when it contracts, it widens the pupil. It is innervated by the sympathetic branch of the autonomic nervous system. The sphincter is the circular muscle at the pupillary margin that constricts the pupil (miosis) when it contracts. It is innervated by the parasympathetic branch of the autonomic nervous system. In addition to light, other factors that affect pupil size include accommodation, injury, disease, age, and refractive error.

Light regulates pupil function by sending a message to the brain (the afferent pathway), which then signals the nervous system (the efferent pathway) to alter the size of the pupil. Light received by the retinal photoreceptor cells stimulates pupillary nerve fibers, which travel with the visual nerve fibers through the optic nerve. The pupillary fibers cross at the chiasm and continue posteriorly into the optic tracts (Figure 5-3). However, they part company with the visual fibers before the lateral geniculate body and travel medially through the brain to a location in the midbrain called the *pretectal nucleus*. After synapsing there, the fibers enter the Edinger-Westphal nucleus of the IIIN (oculomotor nerve) nuclear complex.

Temporal pupillary fibers enter this nucleus ipsilateral (on the same side) to the eyes from which they came; nasal pupillary fibers enter the nucleus contralateral (on the opposite side) to their origins. This is how the brain regulates the 2 pupils equally. This equal constriction is called the *consensual response*. The parasympathetic efferent pathway away from the Edinger-Westphal nucleus follows the third nerve anteriorly to the ciliary ganglion located in the lateral aspect of the posterior orbit. After synapsing there, the fibers enter the eye to innervate the sphincter muscle to constrict the pupil. Pupillary constriction as a response to light stimulation is called the *direct response*.

The dilator muscle is stimulated to contract under conditions of low illumination, when the visual system wants more light, as well as under conditions of physical or emotional stress. It is regulated by the sympathetic nervous system, which is also responsible for the body's fight or flight response—increased heart rate and perspiration, decreased peripheral blood flow, dilated pupils, etc. The efferent system for the pupil dilator muscle begins in the hypothalamus, with 3 sequential neurons that travel down the cervical spine, over the tops of the lungs, and back up the neck to the eyes.

Examination of the pupils with a light stimulus provides evidence of the health of both the afferent and efferent systems. In addition to light, the pupils also respond to accommodation and convergence for clear and single vision at near. The pupils will constrict equally when either accommodation or convergence is stimulated by a near object. When all 3 actions—accommodation, convergence, and miosis—occur simultaneously, this is called the *synkinetic near response*.

Examining the Pupil

OptA

OphA

Pupil function is evaluated with a bright penlight or other intense, small light in a dimly illuminated room. Pupil or iris abnormalities found with the naked eye can then be more thoroughly evaluated using the biomicroscope. The pupils are evaluated for size, shape, direct light response, consensual response, and near response.

What the Patient Needs to Know

- Keep both eyes open during the test.
- Do not look directly at the light.
- Continue to look at the target during the exam.

Size

In dim illumination, the average pupil diameter is 3 or 4 mm. This is ascertained by shining the light from below the patient's nose so that the pupils are just visible to the examiner; the light is not shone directly into the patient's eye. The assistant can then use a millimeter rule (or the half circles printed on the bottom of a near card) to measure the pupil diameters. With experience, the assistant will become fairly accurate at estimating this measurement at a glance. Pupils smaller than 2 mm are said to be miotic; pupils larger than 6 mm are mydriatic. Miotic pupils may be caused by antiglaucoma medications, chronic iris inflammation, age, or a neurologic disorder. Mydriatic pupils are normally more common in children, myopic eyes, and in eyes with a light-colored iris. Abnormal mydriasis is caused by certain drugs, neurologic disorders, iris injury, or acute glaucoma.

The pupils should be equal in size, although a small difference (1 mm) may be a normal variation. If they are unequal (anisocoria), the difference between them should be further evaluated in both dark and bright room illumination. If the difference is greater in dark illumination, then it is likely that the dilator muscle of the eye with the smaller pupil is not working properly. If the difference is greater in light illumination, when the pupils should be relatively miotic, the sphincter muscle of the larger pupil is probably at fault. This is a quick method of deciding whether the problem lies with the sympathetic versus the parasympathetic system. If one pupil remains the same size in light and dark conditions, the iris muscles themselves may have been affected by trauma or drugs (including some eyedrops). When one or both pupils are fully dilated and nonreactive (blown pupils), the assistant must consider this an emergency after ascertaining that drugs or previous injury are not the cause. Nonreactive pupils may be caused by severe head injury or a hemorrhage in the brain, among other things.

Shape

Both pupils should be round. The pupils are normally centered or a little nasal in the iris. An eccentric pupil may be the result of faulty embryonic development, injury, intraocular surgery, or inflammation. In addition to being eccentric, a pupil may also have an unusual shape. Prior surgery or injury may have left scar tissue that has contracted and pulled a section of the pupil margin away from its normal position. This pupil abnormality is called a *peaked pupil* (Figure 6-1) and usually does not affect the patient's visual function. Chronic inflammation can cause loss of stromal tissue of the iris. Tissue loss at the pupillary margin is irregular and makes

Figure 6-1. An abnormal pupil shape may be the result of surgery. (Courtesy of Dennis Ryll.) (Reprinted from Herrin MP. *Ophthalmic Examination and Basic Skills.* Thorofare, NJ: SLACK Incorporated; 1990.)

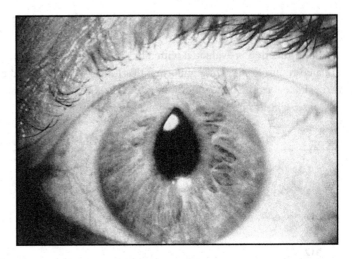

the normally round pupil appear to be scalloped. This appearance may also be caused by sections of the iris margin adhering to the anterior lens capsule (posterior synechiae). The haptics of some iris-fixated intraocular lenses (IOLs) make the iris look square. The assistant should check with the doctor before instilling dilating drops in eyes with these or some anterior chamber IOLs.

Near Response

Pupil response to a near stimulus can be elicited separately or in conjunction with the light response. When testing separately, the assistant holds a near target in front of the eyes, about 12 in from the bridge of the nose. While observing the patient's pupils, the assistant instructs the patient to shift his or her view from a distant target to the near one. The pupils should constrict briskly. The near response can also be checked after the direct light examination, using the light source as a near target. In this instance, the normal pupils should remain at least as small as they were under direct light stimulation. Because there is only one instance where the light response and near response differ (Argyll-Robertson pupil, discussed next), it is not necessary to test the near reaction if the light reaction is intact.

Direct Light Response

In dim room illumination, the patient is instructed to look at a distant target (this prevents the pupillary response to a near stimulus). The light source is presented to each eye separately and slightly off center to avoid the near response (Figure 6-2). Each pupil should exhibit a brisk response and constrict to about 2 mm. If the light is held in front of an eye for a few seconds, the assistant may note that the pupil is constantly moving, alternately constricting and slightly dilating. This phenomenon is called *hippus* and represents the normal condition of maintaining equilibrium between the opposing muscles of the pupil. While shining the light in one eye, the assistant can quickly check the unstimulated pupil for a consensual response (ie, equal constriction). The light response is recorded as an estimation of briskness on a scale of 1 to 4, with 4 being the most brisk. Some examiners also record the change in pupil size with the light response (LR).

Example: 4 mm / round / 3+ LR (or 4 - 2 mm, etc)

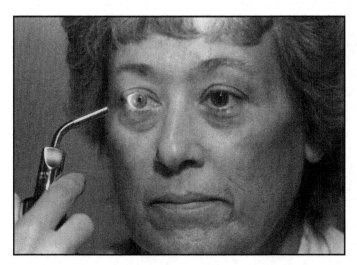

Figure 6-2. Shine the light from the side when testing the direct light response. (Photo by Mark Arrigoni.) (Reprinted from Herrin MP. *Ophthalmic Examination and Basic Skills*. Thorofare, NJ: SLACK Incorporated; 1990.)

Consensual Response

The consensual response is the simultaneous and equal response of one pupil when the other pupil is being stimulated by direct illumination or a near target. If the stimulated pupil constricts normally, then the consensual response of the other pupil will produce equal constriction without direct light stimulus. If the stimulated pupil does not demonstrate full constriction to direct light, then, by consensual response, the other pupil will not fully constrict either. The consensual response is due to the cross-innervation of the afferent system described earlier in this chapter.

Testing the Afferent System

A defect in the afferent system means that the signal being carried from the eye to the brain has been interrupted. This interruption can be partial or complete and can occur anywhere in the visual system where one eye might be affected more than the other (ie, more anterior in the system). The normal eye will exhibit the usual brisk response, while the problematic eye will have a diminished response. This condition, relative afferent pupillary defect (RAPD), is best observed using the swinging flashlight test. The test is performed as follows:

1. The light is presented to one eye, and its direct response is noted.
2. The light is quickly moved across the bridge of the nose to the other eye. There should be little or no constriction of the second pupil because it is already consensually constricted. However, the second pupil may dilate or constrict relative to the first pupil under the following conditions:
   - If the first pupil constricts little or not at all and the second pupil constricts to direct stimulation, then there is an afferent problem in the first eye. With the second eye constricted to the light stimulus, the first eye's pupil should now be consensually constricted.
   - If the first pupil constricts fully and the second pupil dilates to direct stimulation, then the second eye has a RAPD and had been constricted consensually. The first pupil will now be relatively dilated in consensual response with the defective pupil.

This RAPD is demonstrated by moving the light source rapidly back and forth between the 2 eyes and noting each pupil's response relative to the other (Figure 6-3). The pupil that dilates with

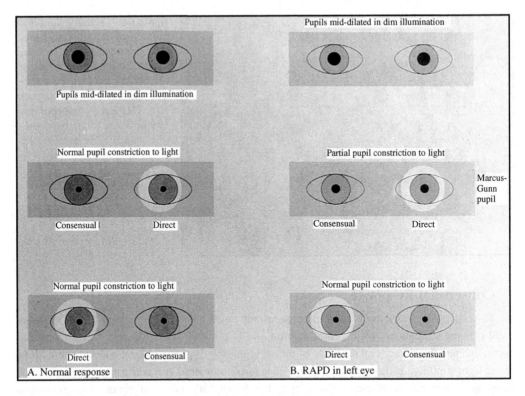

Figure 6-3. Pupil function. (A) Normal direct and consensual response to light stimulation. (B) Abnormal direct response (RAPD or Marcus-Gunn pupil) of the left eye. (Reprinted from Cassin B, Hamed LM, eds. *Fundamentals for Ophthalmic Technical Personnel.* Philadelphia, Pa: WB Saunders Co; 1995.)

direct stimulation has an afferent defect relative to the other pupil. Both pupils may have an afferent problem, but they are usually asymmetric, and a RAPD can be elicited in the more affected eye.

The RAPD is also called the *Marcus-Gunn pupil,* named for the person who first described the paradoxic dilation of the pupil to a light stimulus.

It is sometimes difficult to appreciate a subtle RAPD or to evaluate the pupils of dark-eyed individuals in general. The assistant can dim the room lights completely and use a very bright light (eg, the indirect ophthalmoscope [Figure 6-4]) to improve examination conditions. Another option is to view the suspected problem pupil with a slit lamp. First, the slit lamp is positioned to focus on the pupil, and the patient is instructed to look past the examiner. Then, the slit beam is turned all the way down, and a penlight is shone in the unobserved eye. Next, the penlight is moved away and the slit beam is turned all the way up as the assistant observes whether there is paradoxic dilation. This requires a little practice but gives a magnified view of the pupil in question.

If there is any doubt about the presence of a RAPD, the assistant should ask the doctor to confirm or deny the finding before any drops are instilled.

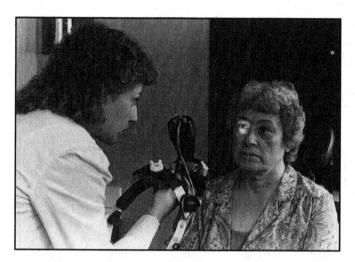

Figure 6-4. The indirect ophthalmoscope can provide a very bright light when testing a questionable Marcus-Gunn pupillary response. (Photo by Mark Arrigoni.) (Reprinted from Herrin MP. *Ophthalmic Examination and Basic Skills.* Thorofare, NJ: SLACK Incorporated; 1990.)

The Efferent System

When the signal going to the brain from the eyes is intact, yet the pupils do not react appropriately, the problem is probably in the efferent system that regulates pupil response. The parasympathetic fibers governing the sphincter muscle travel with the oculomotor nerve to the ciliary ganglion in the posterior orbit and then to the pupil. The sympathetic pathway to the dilator muscle is largely located in the neck and upper chest cavity, derived from the ophthalmic branch of the trigeminal nerve.

Lesions affecting the ciliary ganglion may create a pupillary abnormality called an *Adie's* or *tonic pupil*. There is reduced input to the sphincter, which makes the pupil initially appear larger than the unaffected pupil. Different parts of the sphincter have different degrees of denervation, causing the pupil to have a slow, undulating movement during constriction. Once constricted, the pupil is slow to redilate. Eventually, the pupil may remain in this miotic state. The tonic pupil is part of a syndrome that most often occurs in young women and may have resulted from a viral infection. In 90% of people with an Adie's pupil, there is also loss of deep tendon reflexes.

The dilator function can be impaired by damage to any of the 3 neurons that innervate it. When the dilator is not functioning normally, the affected pupil will be miotic relative to the other one. Light, near, and consensual responses are not affected. The difference between the 2 pupil sizes will be more pronounced in the dark (which is when the dilator is primarily responsible for pupil size.) Miosis produced by a sympathetic system problem has associated physical findings that are also governed by the sympathetic system. One of these is lid ptosis due to denervation of the accessory Mueller's muscle, and the other is lack of sweating (anhidrosis) on the same side of the face. This constellation of signs is called *Horner's syndrome*, and the nerve damage may have been caused by injury, disease, or vascular problems. Congenital Horner's syndrome is a benign condition probably caused by a birth injury or viral infection during infancy and is characterized by having a lighter colored iris than the unaffected eye (heterochromia). Acquired Horner's syndrome may require further investigation because a life-threatening disease may be the cause of the nerve defect.

Finally, there is a central nervous system disorder that affects both pupils; the disorder may be caused by diabetes or alcoholism and (less frequently) by tertiary syphilis. The pupils are small, unequal in size, and irregularly shaped. The condition is called *Argyll-Robertson pupil* and

Table 6-1
Characteristics of Pupillary Disorders

	Size	Shape	Light Rx*	Consensual	Near Rx*
Afferent					
Marcus Gunn	Normal	Normal	Dilation	Normal	Normal
Efferent					
A. Parasympathetic					
III N Palsy	Widely Dilated	Normal	None	None	None
Adie's pupil	Dilated	Irregular	Slow	Slow	Gradual/slow
Argyll-Robertson pupil	Miotic	Irregular	None	None	Normal
B. Sympathetic					
Horner's syndrome	Miotic	Normal	Normal	Normal	Normal
Other					
Physiologic anisocoria	Unequal	Normal	Normal	Normal	Normal
Fixed pupil (amaurotic)	Dilated	Round/oval	None	None	None

* Rx = reaction

is recognizable by the dissociation of light and near responses. Neither pupil reacts to light stimulus, but both have a near response. This is a situation where it is important to observe both light and near responses. If neither pupil reacts to light, then the near response must be tested.

    Example: OD 2 mm / irregular / 1+ LR / 3+ NR
                         2 mm / irregular / 1+ LR / 3+ NR   no RAPD

Hallmarks of Pupil Dysfunction

Table 6-1 compares the findings associated with different pupil disorders.

Chapter 7

Interpupillary Distance, Near Point of Accommodation, and Near Point of Convergence

KEY POINTS

- Be careful not to introduce parallax when measuring IPD.

- The near point of accommodation (NPA) is a monocular test of both eyes.

- The NPA is measured with the patient wearing distance correction.

- An eye that has undergone cataract extraction has no accommodative ability.

- The near point of convergence (NPC) is a binocular test.

- Determine if the patient can appreciate diplopia before attempting the NPC test.

Interpupillary Distance

Accurate measurement of the IPD is important for the correct placement of the OCs of spectacle lenses. As described in Chapter 3, incorrectly placed OCs result in induced prism, which in turn stimulates an extraocular muscle imbalance that may be symptomatic. The amount of prism induced is directly proportional to the power of the lens, so correct OC placement is more critical in higher powered lenses.

When viewing a distant target, the eyes are essentially parallel. The average IPD in adults is about 60 mm and in children about 50 mm. When viewing a near target, the eyes converge, and the IPD decreases by about 3 mm. The closer the object, the smaller the IPD for a given individual. The IPD recorded for spectacles is the distance measurement.

The IPD is measured using the corneal light reflex or by using the corneal limbus as a landmark. Both methods require that the examiner close one eye to avoid an inaccuracy induced by parallax. Also, once the examiner's eye and the patient's eye are aligned for the measurement, neither should move his or her head.

The Corneal Reflex Measurement

The examiner sits directly in front of the patient, closes the right eye, and has the patient look at the open left eye. This essentially places the patient's eye in the straight ahead position. A millimeter rule is placed across the bridge of the patient's nose just under the pupils. The examiner then shines a light into the patient's right eye from just under or beside his or her own left eye and places the zero mark of the ruler precisely below the corneal light reflection (Figure 7-1). Without moving the ruler, the examiner closes the left eye and opens the right eye. Asking the patient to shift fixation to the open eye, the examiner moves the light source to the other side. The examiner then notes the mark on the ruler where the light reflection falls on the patient's left cornea. This number is generally recorded in millimeters, although the calculation used to determine the amount of induced prism uses this number in centimeter form.

If the patient is monocular, the IPD can be measured from the bridge of the nose instead of from the other eye. It should be noted that the bifocal segment does not have to be set more nasally in a monocular patient because the patient will read with one eye only; this does not require convergence.

The Corneal Limbus Measurement

This method is similar to the corneal reflection method. The patient uses the examiner's open eye (first the left, then the right) as alternating targets. Instead of the light reflection, the examiner lines up the zero mark on the ruler with the temporal limbus of the patient's right eye (Figure 7-2). After switching fixation, the examiner notes where the ruler mark falls relative to the patient's left nasal limbus. This is a very convenient method for measuring near IPD because the examiner's open left eye serves as a near target for the patient's open eyes. As the patient continues to look at the examiner's open left eye, the examiner sets the zero mark at the patient's right temporal limbus. Then, without moving, and using the left eye, the examiner notes the ruler mark that is directly beneath the patient's left nasal limbus.

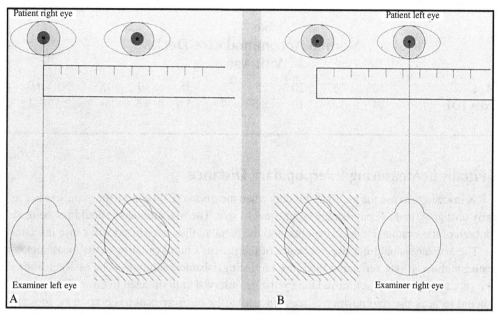

Figure 7-1. View to pupil. Distance IPD using the corneal light reflex. (A) The examiner's left eye views the patient's right eye and sets the zero mark. Without moving, the examiner's right eye then views the patient's left eye (B) and notes the mark on the ruler. (Reprinted from Cassin B, Hamed LM, eds. *Fundamentals of Ophthalmic Technical Personnel*. Philadelphia, Pa: WB Saunders Co; 1995.)

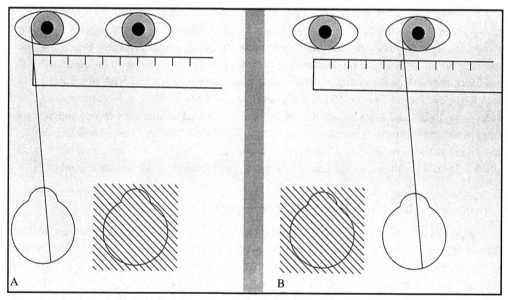

Figure 7-2. View to limbus. Distance IPD using the patient's (A) right corneal limbus and (B) left nasal limbus. (Reprinted from Cassin B, Hamed LM, eds. *Fundamentals of Ophthalmic Technical Personnel*. Philadelphia, Pa: WB Saunders Co; 1995.)

Table 7-1 Normal Accommodative Decline With Age										
Age	5	10	15	20	25	30	35	40	45	50	60
NPA (D)	16	14	12	10	8.5	7	5.5	4.5	4	2.5	1

Pitfalls in Measuring Interpupillary Distance

It is inaccurate to use the pupillary borders when measuring IPD because the pupil size is constantly changing, and the pupils may be unequal in size. The measurements should not be made with both of the examiner's eyes open because the parallax thus introduced will cause inaccuracies. The assistant should not use the center of the patient's pupil to estimate the measurement, because without a light reflection there are no distinguishable landmarks. The assistant should make sure the patient has not moved the eye being observed until directed to do so. The examiner should recheck the zero position at least once after the measurement has been made to verify the starting point.

Near Point of Accommodation

Measuring near point of accommodation (NPA) is a monocular test of the eye's ability to maintain clear focus on a near object. It is defined as the closest point that a target is seen clearly and represents the maximum accommodation that the eye can naturally exert. Because accommodation is a function of the performance of the ciliary muscle coupled with the elasticity of the lens itself, the NPA and accommodative reserve diminish with age. The NPA of a child is very close to the eye (about 7 cm or 15 D), while a 60-year-old adult's NPA is 50 cm or more (≤2 D) (Table 7-1). Decreased accommodative ability is often noticed around 40 years of age and continues to diminish. If there is no natural lens in the eye, as after cataract extraction or lens replacement, there is no accommodation at all. Also, accommodation may be nonexistent if the ciliary muscle has been paralyzed or the central nervous system control center has been damaged.

Measuring the Near Point of Accommodation

The patient must be wearing his or her full distance correction; the bifocal should not be used. The patient is instructed to cover one eye and look at an accommodative target (no larger than 20/40 size on a near card). The target is moved slowly toward the patient's open eye (Figure 7-3) until the patient reports that the target is no longer clear. This point is the NPA and is measured from the cornea to the target at the blur point. The NPA may be recorded in centimeters or diopters, which are easily interchanged (D = 100 / NPA in cm). The Prince rule, a bar ruler often attached to the front of the phoropter, has both metric and dioptric markings.

The NPA should be about the same for each eye, assuming that the natural lens is present in both eyes. If the NPA is significantly unequal, the assistant should recheck the distance correction for an undiscovered refractive error in one eye. The inequity may be due to monocular damage to the accommodative system or some disease process, so it is important to accurately

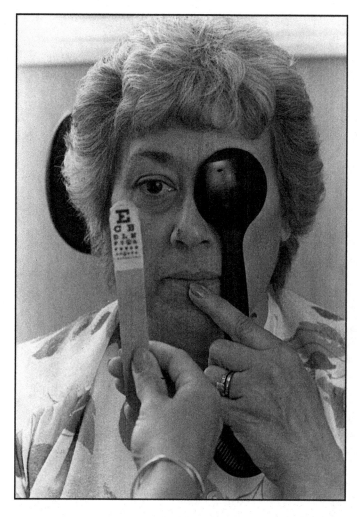

Figure 7-3. An accommodative target is moved toward the eye. The patient is asked to state when the target is no longer clearly seen. (Photo by Mark Arrigoni.) (Reprinted from Herrin MP. *Ophthalmic Examination and Basic Skills.* Thorofare, NJ: SLACK Incorporated; 1990.)

document any inequality. The assistant must remember that an eye that has undergone cataract extraction has no accommodative ability.

The NPA is no longer obtainable once the pupils have been dilated, so the assistant must be sure to do these measurements, if indicated, before dilating drops have been instilled. Occasionally, accommodation may be so low that the NPA is too remote for the patient to be able to distinguish the target. In this instance, the assistant can place a plus lens over the distance correction that is just strong enough to make the target clear at arm's length. The NPA is measured in the same manner as previously described, but the amount of the added plus lens must then be subtracted from the final dioptric NPA.

Near Point of Convergence

As noted previously, the eyes are essentially parallel when viewing a distant object. In order to maintain the image of a near object on both foveas, the eyes must converge (ie, move toward the midline). The nearer the object, the more convergence must be exerted to maintain single vision. The closest point at which the eyes can maintain single vision by exerting maximum con-

Figure 7-4. A target is slowly moved at eye level toward the bridge of the patient's nose. (Photo by Mark Arrigoni.) (Reprinted from Herrin MP. *Ophthalmic Examination and Basic Skills.* Thorofare, NJ: SLACK Incorporated; 1990.)

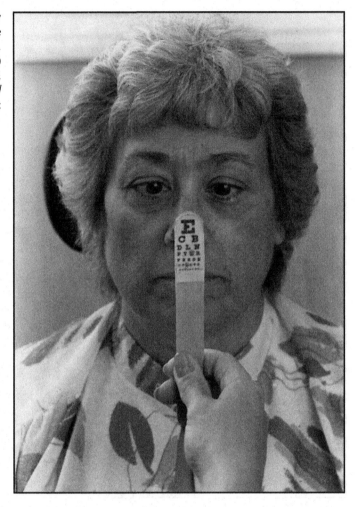

vergence is called the *Near Point of Convergence* (NPC). In young people, the NPC may be as close as the nose, but, as with accommodation, the point becomes more remote with age (although not to the same extent). At some point, a remote NPC may cause symptoms of eyestrain, headaches, etc.

Measuring the Near Point of Convergence

This test differs from the NPA in that it is a test of binocular function and requires both eyes to be open. The target is moved slowly toward the bridge of the patient's nose (Figure 7-4). The patient is instructed to maintain fixation on the approaching target, to report first when the target becomes blurred (the endpoint of accommodative convergence), and then when the target becomes double. The nearest point where the target is still single, the NPC, is measured in centimeters. The normal value for children is 5 to 10 cm, but adults may have an NPC more remote than 10 cm. In some patients with convergence insufficiency, the NPC may exceed 25 cm.

Sometimes, the patient will not be able to appreciate double vision or cannot distinguish between a blurred image and a double image. The assistant, who is observing the patient's eyes throughout this test, will observe the eyes moving toward each other and will notice when convergence breaks. As the eyes reach and then exceed maximum convergence, one eye will drift outward. This point is a reasonable objective estimation of the NPC.

Insufficient convergence is frequently seen in young adults whose reading or other near vision demands suddenly increase. A remote NPC and/or insufficient convergence reserves may lead to asthenopic symptoms. Convergence exercises, prescribed and monitored by an eyecare professional, are generally highly effective in improving convergence function and relieving symptoms. For more details, please consult the Series title *A Systematic Approach to Strabismus*.

What the Patient Needs to Know

- Continue to look at the target as instructed.

- Do not use your bifocal or reading glasses.

- Let the assistant know if you are confused about what to do.

Chapter 8

The Slit Lamp Exam

- Make sure the patient is comfortable for the exam.
- Keep the light just bright enough to do the exam.
- Develop a systematic way to do a complete, efficient exam.

The slit lamp is the common name for the biomicroscope, a binocular microscope that has been designed to give a magnified view of the anterior segment of the eye in the examining room. The slit lamp is equipped with a movable light source, variable beam dimension, at least 2 magnifications, and chin and forehead rests for the patient. The lid skin and margins can be examined under lower magnification, while the corneal layers, anterior chamber, iris features, and lens details are more visible under higher magnification. In addition to the internal magnification lenses, there may be an attached Hruby lens, which allows a restricted but highly magnified view of the vitreous and retina. Also attached to the slit lamp is a tonometer for measuring intraocular pressure (IOP). For a full discussion of the slit lamp, please consult the Series title *The Slit Lamp Primer*, 2nd edition.

Using the Slit Lamp

The slit lamp is usually situated on a movable arm of the instrument stand beside the exam chair. The arm can be moved toward the seated patient so that the slit lamp table is at about waist level, and the patient can rest his or her head comfortably on the chin rest. The instrument should not be so high that the patient has to stretch his or her neck or so low that the patient is bent over and cannot use the chin rest (Figure 8-1). The slit lamp table can be moved up or down, and the patient's chair height can be adjusted to accommodate the patient's stature. In addition, the instrument must be close enough so that the patient's head will remain firmly against the forehead rest during the exam. If the patient's head drifts back, the examiner may not be able to maintain focus. Once the patient's head is positioned, the chin rest is adjusted so that the lateral canthi are aligned with the mark on the side bars. The patient's eyes can be positioned as needed by instructing him or her to view appropriate targets with the eye not being examined. The patient should be encouraged and reminded to blink normally.

Preparing the Instrument

The 2 oculars on the slit lamp must be set for both the examiner's IPD and refractive error. While looking through both oculars, the assistant moves the oculars either closer together or farther apart to get a clear and unobstructed view. Then, the 2 oculars are adjusted for focus. If the assistant is wearing spectacles or contact lenses, the oculars are focused near zero. If correction is not worn, the refractive correction can be dialed in on the oculars themselves. This adjustment is important for obtaining a clear view, but over-minusing is not an issue (as with the keratometer or lensometer) because no measurements are being made.

The range of available magnification varies according to the instrument. The Haag-Streit slit lamp (Figure 8-2) features a lever just under the oculars that changes the magnification from low power (1x) to high power (1.6x). More magnification can be obtained by replacing the oculars themselves with higher powered ones. Other types of slit lamps have a dial on the body of the instrument that offers 3 different magnifications. Both the lever and dial are easily accessible and can be used to change the magnification without interrupting the examination. The lower powers are generally used for external exam (lids, conjunctiva, cornea, etc) and for performing tonometry. The higher powers are used for a magnified view of intraocular structures and contents of the anterior chamber.

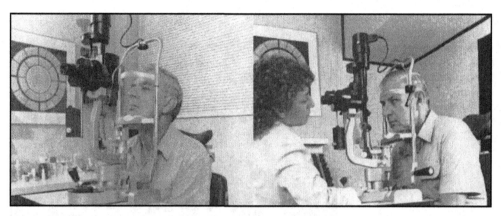

Figure 8-1. (A) The slit lamp is too high for the patient. (B) The slit lamp is too low for the patient. (Photos by Mark Arrigoni.) (Reprinted from Herrin MP. *Ophthalmic Examination and Basic Skills.* Thorofare, NJ: SLACK Incorporated; 1990.)

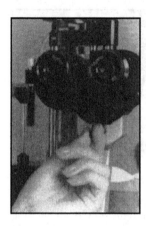

Figure 8-2. Magnification is changed by flipping a lever. Other instruments may have a magnification knob behind the oculars. (Photo by Mark Arrigoni.) (Reprinted from Herrin MP. *Ophthalmic Examination and Basic Skills.* Thorofare, NJ: SLACK Incorporated; 1990.)

The joystick at the base of the instrument moves the entire instrument vertically, horizontally, forward, and backward. The width of the slit beam can be adjusted by the dial at the base of the tower, and the height of the beam is determined by a dial at the top of the tower.

Once the patient is properly positioned, the instrument is turned on, and the magnification is set to low power. The slit lamp is moved toward the patient so that the light is visible on the patient's right eye (Figure 8-3). The features of the eye should now be visible through the oculars. If the patient's eye is not visible, the assistant should check the ocular settings, patient position, and light source position. Once the eye is in focus, the assistant may begin the exam.

What the Patient Needs to Know

- Maintain your position, keeping your chin in the chin rest and head against the bar.

- Let the assistant know if you are uncomfortable.

- Do not talk during the exam; try to keep your head still.

Figure 8-3. The slit beam is visible on the patient's right eye when the instrument is grossly aligned. (Photo by Mark Arrigoni.) (Reprinted from Herrin MP. *Ophthalmic Examination and Basic Skills.* Thorofare, NJ: SLACK Incorporated; 1990.)

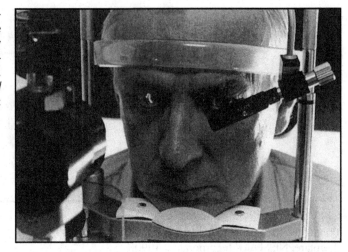

Figure 8-4. (A and B) Diffuse illumination. (Photo by Mark Arrigoni.) (Reprinted from Herrin MP. *Ophthalmic Examination and Basic Skills.* Thorofare, NJ: SLACK Incorporated; 1990.)

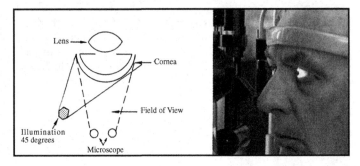

Smooth, efficient use of the slit lamp comes with practice, and the assistant will become adept at using both hands simultaneously to move the instrument, adjust the light source, change the magnification, hold the lids open, etc. The assistant should be gentle and considerate of the patient at all times. The assistant should keep in mind that his or her job is to detect and document any abnormalities, not to make a diagnosis or discuss findings with the patient.

Types of Illumination

The light source and viewing angle can be adjusted relative to each other to allow a view of different parts of the anterior segment that would not otherwise be visible. Various illumination techniques are discussed briefly here.

Direct diffuse illumination (Figure 8-4) permits a direct view of a broad section of the external structures, cornea, and iris. The beam is at full width, and the light source is moved to about 45 degrees from the microscope. The light intensity should be just bright enough to do the examination but not so bright as to cause the patient discomfort.

Direct focal illumination (Figure 8-5) uses a very narrow beam directed from 45 degrees. This angle and slit lamp position sends the beam past the pupil margin and through the lens so that there is no reflection from an internal surface. This technique allows a view of the corneal surface and anterior layers. Parallelipiped illumination uses a slightly broader beam than the direct focal and is used to view a cross section of the cornea and endothelium. When the slit lamp is

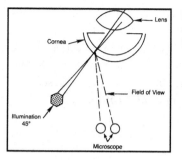

Figure 8-5. Direct focal illumination. (Reprinted from Herrin MP. *Ophthalmic Examination and Basic Skills.* Thorofare, NJ: SLACK Incorporated; 1990.)

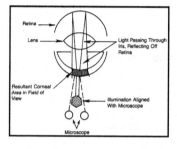

Figure 8-6. Retroillumination. (Reprinted from Herrin MP. *Ophthalmic Examination and Basic Skills.* Thorofare, NJ: SLACK Incorporated; 1990.)

moved peripherally and the focus is shifted posteriorly, the iris is clearly visible. In this case, the slit beam is directed at the iris, not past it, in what is called *tangential illumination.*

Scleral scatter illumination is used to visualize abnormalities of the cornea that are not visible with direct illumination. A narrow beam is directed at the temporal limbus and reflected internally to detail changes that are usually transparent.

Finally, the light may be moved to a position directly in front of the microscope so the beam is aimed through the pupil and lens to the retina. The light reflected back to the viewer from the retina is called *retroillumination* (Figure 8-6) and is used to visualize certain structures or abnormalities of the lens, iris, or cornea.

Examination of the Anterior Segment

OphA

Cornea

CL

The cornea—the clear, refracting surface at the most anterior aspect of the eye—is about 0.5 mm thick and is made up of 5 layers. The outermost layer, the epithelium, is about 5 cell layers thick and serves both as a protective barrier and as the regulator of stromal hydration. The basement membrane of the epithelial cells lies against the second corneal layer, Bowman's layer (also called *Bowman's membrane*, although not a true membrane), which is an acellular region of the anterior stroma. The third layer, the stroma, is the thickest part of the cornea, constituting 90% of corneal tissue. The precise lamellar arrangement of the stromal cells and their specific level of hydration account for the transparency of the cornea. The fourth layer is Descemet's membrane, the basement membrane for the internal endothelium layer. Descemet's membrane serves as a barrier to the influx of water from the anterior chamber while the endothelial cells actively pump water out of the stroma. Corneal anatomy and physiology are covered in more detail in the Series title *Ocular Anatomy and Physiology.*

Using diffuse, low-level illumination, the cornea is first examined for gross abnormalities, such as scars, and surface irregularities. Then, using the slit beam for direct focal illumination, the different layers of the cornea can be evaluated either individually or in cross section. In particular, the entire cornea should be smooth, glistening, and completely transparent. The following is a list of more common corneal abnormalities seen with the slit lamp. A detailed description of corneal pathology may be found in the Series title *Overview of Ocular Disorders.*

Opacities

- Scars left by trauma, infection, etc.
- Mineral deposits associated with different diseases, metabolic or environmental conditions, structural changes, etc.
- Metabolic deposition (eg, lipids as in arcus senilis).
- Endothelial deposits of pigment or inflammatory cells (keratic precipitates).
- Embedded foreign bodies (eg, wood, metal, etc).

Haze

- Stromal damage after infection, excimer laser treatment, trauma, etc.
- Extensive epithelial keratopathy.
- Edema caused by disruption of the endothelium.
- Endothelial stippling due to guttata, dystrophies, etc.

Vascularization

- Fine blood vessels at the limbus (pannus).
- Larger vascular "trees" growing toward central scars or active pathology.

Surface Irregularities

- Epithelial punctate keratopathy due to dryness, irritation, or infection.
- Corneal ulcers, larger areas of epithelial or stromal loss.
- Recurrent erosions in which small areas of epithelium are easily and repeatedly dislodged.

Some dystrophies or other endothelial changes are best visualized using retroillumination. Also, epithelial changes may be seen in more detail using special stains for diseased (rose bengal) or dead (fluorescein) cells. These stains are discussed in Chapter 1.

Some slit lamps have an attached pachymeter for estimating the thickness of the cornea. The slit beam is turned horizontally, and the length of the beam is adjusted to correspond to the thickness of the cornea. The measurement is read from a dial at the top of the light tower.

The Iris

The colored iris, pale blue to dark brown, is composed of several layers of tissue, including the pupil muscles. Only the anterior surface of the iris is visible, but surface lesions, abnormal blood vessels, or structural changes are readily visualized. Some individuals have fairly smooth iris surfaces, while others have beautifully complex irides featuring crypts and ridges. The iris should be examined for unusual pigment patches that may be normal for the patient; benign nevi (freckles) may also be seen. These pigmented areas rarely represent malignant tumors. Diffuse illumination may be used to grossly identify iris landmarks, and then a tangential slit beam may

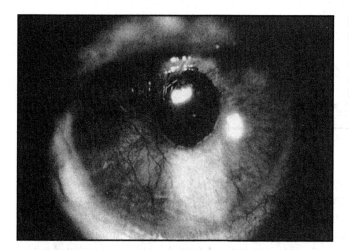

Figure 8-7. A patient with rubeosis iridis. (Courtesy of Dennis Ryll.) (Reprinted from Herrin MP. *Ophthalmic Examination and Basic Skills.* Thorofare, NJ: SLACK Incorporated; 1990.)

be used to visualize detail. The slit beam can also be used to discover and estimate the height of raised lesions on the surface or in the iris stroma.

Another abnormality of the iris is the presence of unusual blood vessels on the surface (Figure 8-7). These neovascular networks are caused by diabetes or follow retinal vessel occlusion; the condition is called *rubeosis iridis.* This type of vasculature does not have the same integrity as normal vessels and can produce glaucoma as well as hemorrhages in the anterior chamber. These new vessels are usually first seen at either the pupillary margin or in the angle (using gonioscopy).

Inflammation of the anterior uveal tract, called *iritis* or *anterior uveitis,* may produce changes in the iris tissue over time or with recurrences. Iris detail may be lost, and iris tissue may adhere to contiguous structures in the eye. In the angle, the iris can become stuck to the corneal endothelium (peripheral anterior synechiae), blocking aqueous outflow. The pupil margin can adhere to the anterior lens capsule (posterior synechiae), blocking aqueous flow from the posterior chamber into the anterior chamber. Both types of synechiae, if extensive enough, may cause secondary glaucoma.

Another type of glaucoma is caused by iris stromal pigment blocking the angle. With the motion of accommodation, lens zonules may rub the back of the iris, dispersing pigment cells into the anterior chamber. They may be seen as a vertical collection on the back of the cornea (Krukenberg's spindle) or in the angle using gonioscopy. With retroillumination, radial spokes of orange light reflected from the retina through the iris may be seen where the pigment cells have been lost.

The Anterior Chamber

Between the posterior cornea and the anterior iris is the anterior chamber, a space filled with the aqueous secreted by the ciliary body. A primary goal of the slit lamp exam is to evaluate the depth of the chamber prior to dilating the pupil. A shallow chamber means that the iris/cornea angle is small and may be occluded by peripheral iris tissue during dilation, causing a rise in IOP. When the slit beam is directed onto the peripheral iris from about 60 degrees, the space between the corneal reflection and the iris reflection can be observed. It appears as a dark band between the light bands on the cornea and iris (Figure 8-8). A deep chamber or wide angle will have a dark band that is at least one-third of the width of the corneal light band. A shallow

Figure 8-8. The difference in the width of the slit lamp will help determine the depth of the anterior chamber. (Drawing by Edmund Pett.) (Reprinted from Herrin MP. *Ophthalmic Examination and Basic Skills.* Thorofare, NJ: SLACK Incorporated; 1990.)

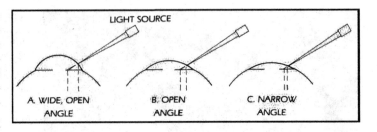

chamber or narrow angle has a thin dark band that is less than one-quarter of the corneal light band width. Occasionally, the angle will be so narrow that the dark band is not appreciable. These patients may have temporary spikes in their IOP when they are in dim illumination and their pupils dilate. Whenever the angle appears narrow, the pupil should not be dilated before the doctor is consulted.

The fluid in the anterior chamber should be invisible and clear of cells, debris, etc. When the anterior segment is inflamed, protein and white blood cells or pigment cells become suspended in the aqueous. The protein renders the normally clear fluid somewhat hazy, a finding called *flare*. Flare can best be appreciated by focusing the microscope in the anterior chamber while a small round bright beam is directed into the chamber from about 45 degrees. In addition to the haze produced by protein, the assistant may also observe cells in the chamber. These look like dust particles floating in a sunbeam and may be yellow (red blood cells), white (white blood cells), or brown (iris pigment cells). These cells are usually seen moving upward along with aqueous flow but may be stationary in a stagnant chamber filled with protein. White or red blood cells may settle at the bottom of the chamber due to gravity; the pool of white cells is called a *hypopyon*, and the red cell pool is a *hyphema*.

The Lens

The lens is a clear, avascular, multilayer structure. It has 2 convex sides and is suspended behind the iris in the posterior chamber by elastic fibers (zonules). The lens has a central nucleus covered with onionskin-like layers (cortex) and is encased in a membranous lens capsule. Using a narrow slit beam, the front and back of the lens can be defined, and the intermediate cortex and nucleus can be evaluated.

The lens is subject to significant aging changes, most notably cataract formation, which are often readily seen with the slit lamp. A senile cataract has a brown discoloration (brunescence), although advanced cataracts are white. Traumatic cataracts occur at the site of penetration and are an opaque white. Posterior subcapsular cataracts are centrally located just inside the posterior capsule and are best observed using retroillumination.

Loss of the lens, through surgery or trauma, renders the eye aphakic. The examiner may observe the intact vitreous face as a smooth clear surface that bulges slightly forward in the pupil. If the vitreous face has been ruptured or incompletely resected during surgery, it may bulge far enough into the anterior chamber to rest against the corneal endothelium. This may interfere with endothelial function, producing a focal area of corneal haze. More often, the examiner will observe the flat, solid surface of a surgically implanted plastic IOL. The IOL should be examined for centration, position with respect to the iris plane, and the presence of optically significant

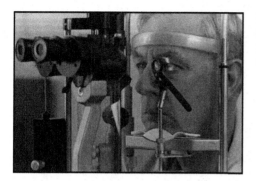

Figure 8-9. Use of the Hruby lens attachment. (Reprinted from Herrin MP. *Ophthalmic Examination and Basic Skills*. Thorofare, NJ: SLACK Incorporated; 1990.)

deposits or scratches. Older IOLs may have been placed in the anterior chamber, but most cataract replacement lenses are now placed in the posterior chamber. Finally, if the posterior capsule remains after IOL implantation, it must be evaluated for visually impairing opacification.

Examination of the Posterior Segment

The Vitreous

The vitreous body is a gelatinous, transparent structure that occupies the large cavity behind the lens. The anterior central portion is visible through the undilated pupil and can be examined for the presence of blood, deposits, or calcification.

The Retina

The Hruby lens is a 55-D plus spherical lens that is used with the slit lamp to view the retinal fundus (Figure 8-9). An extremely limited view is possible through an undilated pupil in a very cooperative patient. The best view is obtained with pupillary dilation using a thin slit beam at a slightly oblique angle. The Hruby lens or a handheld 90-D lens gives a highly magnified, stereoscopic view of the optic nerve, macula, papillomacular nerve fiber bundle, and fundus vasculature. The examiner will be able to observe such abnormalities as optic nerve inflammation or pallor, macular changes, and vascular disorders.

Chapter 9

Tonometry

KEY POINTS

- Tonometry measures intraocular pressure (IOP) in millimeters of mercury.

- Measurement of IOP is vital in diagnosing and monitoring glaucoma.

- Make sure the tonometer is clean and calibrated.

- Repeat any readings that seem unusual.

- Perform tonometry carefully so as not to alarm the patient.

- Wash hands before and after touching the patient.

Intraocular Pressure and Glaucoma

Tonometry is the measurement of intraocular pressure (IOP). By convention, the IOP unit of measurement is millimeters of mercury (mm Hg). The normal range of IOP values is 8 to 21 mm Hg, with higher values indicating the possible presence of the ocular disorder glaucoma. In a normal eye, aqueous is produced by the ciliary body (behind the iris) and is secreted into the posterior chamber. From there, it flows through the pupil into the anterior chamber and exits the eye through the trabecular meshwork of the anterior chamber angle. The delicate balance of aqueous production and outflow is the equilibrium that maintains optimal IOP.

Glaucoma, called "the silent thief of sight," in its most common form is painless as well as insidious in its destruction of the visual field. The disorder is defined by the triad of high IOP, optic nerve damage, and visual field loss. Early detection of glaucoma, usually by routine tonometry, is imperative in halting the progressive loss of vision. Untreated high IOP destroys the nerve fibers in the retina and is most noticeable as tissue loss at the optic disc. The normal (physiologic) cup of the disc, where the nerve fibers and blood vessels exit or enter the eye, is about one-third the size of the whole disc; this is written as a *cup-to-disc (c/d) ratio* of 0.3. When glaucomatous damage occurs, disc tissue loss can be almost complete, with c/d ratios approaching 0.99.

There are several types of glaucoma. The most common type, progressive or chronic open-angle glaucoma, is characterized by a seemingly normal outflow system and overproduction of aqueous. Medical and surgical treatment of this type of glaucoma aims to decrease aqueous production and/or increase the rate of outflow. Untreated, the IOP tends to run in the 20s and low 30s; this is not usually perceptible to the patient.

Angle-closure, or narrow-angle, glaucoma features a shallow anterior chamber and subsequent obstruction of outflow; aqueous production is generally normal. During normal pupil dilation in low illumination or with the use of dilating drops, the angle may be blocked sufficiently to cause a rapid rise in IOP to a level that results in corneal edema and extreme pain. Acute angle-closure glaucoma is an ocular emergency requiring immediate action. Pharmacologic and osmotic agents are used to try to constrict the pupil and stimulate outflow to lower the IOP. Once the attack has been broken and the eye is relatively quiet, surgery or laser can be used to create an alternative outflow route (peripheral iridectomy or iridotomy). This will prevent any further attacks. Because this type of glaucoma is caused by an anatomic abnormality, it is usually bilateral; the second eye will often be treated prophylactically.

Secondary glaucoma results from some other ocular disorder that usually affects the outflow system. Trauma to the eye can close the angle. An enlarged or displaced lens, or 360 degrees of posterior synechiae, can prevent aqueous egression from the posterior chamber; this is called *pupillary block*. Intraocular blood, pigment cells, or debris can clog the trabecular meshwork, obstructing outflow.

Some people are born with glaucoma in one or both eyes. Because the infant eye is in a growth phase and is very elastic, high IOP causes enlargement of the entire globe. The most apparent sign of congenital glaucoma is an oversized eye (buphthalmos) with a cornea so large that very little sclera is visible. In early childhood, the eye loses its ability to stretch, and internal nerve damage begins to occur, as it does in adult glaucoma. Another cause of visual loss in congenital glaucoma is the amblyopia caused by uncorrected high myopia of the large eye (due to the eye's enlargement). The assistant must document large corneas (more than 11 mm) in children younger than 3 years of age.

Finally, there are 2 less common forms of glaucoma. Low-tension glaucoma occurs in some individuals who demonstrate glaucomatous optic nerve damage and visual field loss in the presence of normal IOP. Conversely, some individuals have IOPs that stay in the 20s yet have no evidence of optic disc or visual field changes. This latter condition is known as *ocular hypertension* (OHT) and is believed to precede glaucoma. These individuals should be closely monitored for early glaucomatous changes or treated medically to prevent the possibility of progression. For a full discussion of the types of glaucomas, please refer to the Series title *Cataract and Glaucoma*.

It should be noted that the IOP measurement could be artificially low if the cornea is thin (<550µm) or high if the cornea is thicker than normal. Glaucoma may be under or over diagnosed if IOP is the only factor considered. Conversion values vary in the current literature, but it may be estimated that IOP will be about 2 mmHg different (lower in thinner corneas, higher in thicker corneas) for every 50 microns of variation in corneal thickness compared to normal.

Types of Tonometry

The most accurate instruments for measuring IOP must touch the eye; the preferred site for this measurement is the central cornea. There are 2 basic types of contact tonometry, the applanation and indentation types, with several instruments in each category. Applanation tonometers flatten a small area of the central cornea and measure the amount of force required to do this (against the internal pressure of the eye). The Goldmann and Mentor Pneumatometer™ are examples of applanation instruments. The Goldmann is the most widely used of all tonometers in the office setting and is the standard of accuracy.

The Schiotz and Mentor Tonopen™ tonometers are the most familiar indentation instruments. Indentation tonometry involves a weighted free-moving plunger that indents rather than flattens the cornea.

Applanation Tonometry

The Goldmann tonometer (Figure 9-1) is attached to a slit lamp and used with the light source and one of the oculars of the microscope. The tonometer itself requires little maintenance, although its calibration must be checked periodically. A calibration bar and attachment are supplied with the instrument.

Checking the Goldmann Calibration

The attachment piece (Figure 9-2) is inserted into the calibration port above the dial on the right side, and the bar is positioned so that the middle etched line is aligned with the attachment calibration line. The dial is then rotated to the zero mark. As the dial nears the zero mark, the tonometer head will tilt slightly. Rotating the dial slightly away from zero will cause the head to move back. The calibration bar is then set to the next line, and the dial is rotated to the 2 gm (20 mm Hg) mark, again causing movement of the tonometer head. Finally, the bar is set at the end line, and the dial is rotated to 6 gm (60 mm Hg). At each calibration point, the tonometer head should rock back and forth within ±1 mm Hg of that point. If it does not, the whole unit must be sent to the manufacturer for recalibration.

Cleaning the Tonometer Head

The applanation head is a plastic cone fitted with a prism; the head is removable for cleaning. The head must be cleaned between each patient to avoid the transmission of infectious organisms.

Figure 9-1. The Goldmann applanation tonometer attached to a slit lamp. (Photo by Mark Arrigoni.) (Reprinted from Herrin MP. *Ophthalmic Examination and Basic Skills*. Thorofare, NJ: SLACK Incorporated; 1990.)

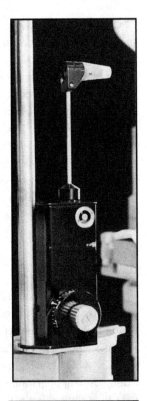

Figure 9-2. Testing the calibration of the Goldmann applanation tonometer. (Photo by Mark Arrigoni.) (Reprinted from Herrin MP. *Ophthalmic Examination and Basic Skills*. Thorofare, NJ: SLACK Incorporated; 1990.)

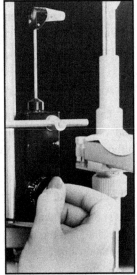

The head can be soaked in 3% hydrogen peroxide or a 1:10 dilution of household bleach for 10 minutes, then rinsed thoroughly with water and blotted dry. No nonrecommended cleaning agents should be used because these can damage the prism or destroy the glue. Some physicians advocate a quick cleaning with an alcohol pad, but the tonometer head must be completely dry before reuse because the alcohol is very injurious to the corneal epithelium. Other physicians criticize this method because a brief wipe with alcohol is not enough to destroy some organisms.

Preparing the Patient

Topical anesthetic and fluorescein dye are used with an applanation tonometer. The drops may be instilled separately, using an appropriate anesthetic (proparacaine, etc) to wet a fluorescein strip or using a drop that combines both. The anesthetic and stain are instilled in the lower fornix of both eyes, and the excess is gently blotted away. The patient is positioned at the slit lamp, and the cornea is briefly checked for any epithelial changes that stain with the fluorescein. The tonometer is then moved into position. Some tonometer attachments are on an arm that swings from the side and clicks into place on a small grooved stage. Other tonometers are at the top of the slit lamp and swing down into the measuring position.

Obtaining the Measurement

With the microscope directed straight ahead, the magnification set low, and the light source set about 60 degrees away, the cobalt blue filter is dialed or flipped into place. To measure the right eye, the patient is instructed to view some straight-ahead target with his or her left eye so that the right eye is properly positioned for applanation. Both eyes should be kept open, and the lids should be relaxed to avoid introducing external pressure to the eye. If the patient is one-eyed or has strabismus, the assistant can verbally direct the patient to move the eye to the correct position. The patient is asked to not move the eyes or head and to keep both eyes open. After a blink to smooth the fluorescein over the corneal surface, the patient should keep both eyes wide open so that the applanator tip does not touch the lid margin or lashes. Often, the lids must be held apart by the assistant, who must take care not to exert any pressure on the eye.

What the Patient Needs to Know

- Breathe normally during this test.

- Keep both eyes open and lids relaxed.

- Do not move your eyes or head during the test.

- Do not be afraid to let the assistant know if you are nervous, uncomfortable, or concerned about the cleanliness of the instruments.

In a smooth, rapid sequence, the tonometer head is positioned in front of and very close to the cornea without touching it. Only one of the oculars gives a view of the prism. The assistant either looks through the left ocular with the right eye or through both oculars with concentration on the eye with the best view of the prism. The assistant will see a blue field with very pale half circles divided horizontally. Looking through the ocular, the assistant slowly and steadily moves the applanator to make gentle contact with the eye (Figure 9-3). As soon as contact is made, the half circles (mires) become bright yellow and distinct (Figure 9-4). The mires should be centered in the field and equal in size. If they are unequal, this indicates that the tonometer is too high (larger circle on the bottom) or too low (larger circle on the top [Figure 9-5]). The slit lamp is pulled back slightly to break contact, and the height is adjusted appropriately.

Once the mires are equalized, they must be correctly positioned relative to each other using the pressure dial. If the mires are completely separated from each other, more pressure must be dialed in until the inner sides of each are just touching each other (Figure 9-6). If the mires overlap without touching each other, the dial is set too high and must be rotated to a lower setting. As soon as the mires are properly aligned, the slit lamp is pulled back, and the number is read

Figure 9-3. Touching the cornea with the applanator head. (Photo by Mark Arrigoni.) (Reprinted from Herrin MP. *Ophthalmic Examination and Basic Skills.* Thorofare, NJ: SLACK Incorporated; 1990.)

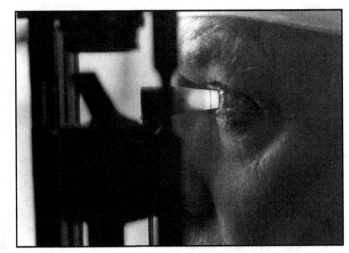

Figure 9-4. The fluorescein breaks into 2 half-circles. (Reprinted from Herrin MP. *Ophthalmic Examination and Basic Skills.* Thorofare, NJ: SLACK Incorporated; 1990.)

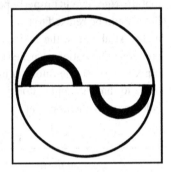

Figure 9-5. The tonometer is too low. (Reprinted from Herrin MP. *Ophthalmic Examination and Basic Skills.* Thorofare, NJ: SLACK Incorporated; 1990.)

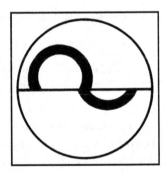

Figure 9-6. The proper position of the circles for pressure measurement.

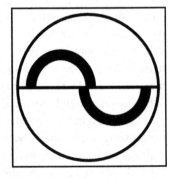

from the dial. This number is multiplied by 10 and recorded as the IOP in mm Hg. A second quick look at the stained cornea will ensure that any applanation-induced epithelial damage will be noted. A faint circular imprint may be visible and is not clinically significant.

The left eye is measured in the same way. If the patient has deep-set eyes, the light source may be moved to the right side of the slit lamp so that the light is not blocked by the bridge of the nose.

Sources of Error

One measurement of each eye is usually sufficient. However, if the patient is being followed for glaucoma or the first measurement is suspect, 2 readings should be taken on each eye.

If the cornea is astigmatic, the mires will not appear as semi-circles and will not align accurately. The tonometer head has degree marks opposite the prism for adjusting the prism position to compensate for more than 3 D of corneal astigmatism. This astigmatism cannot be determined from the spectacles because the cylinder in a prescription may include lenticular astigmatism. It is best to get a keratometric reading of the corneal curvature and use the axis of the greater radius (least dioptric) or minus cylinder axis. This axis mark on the tonometer head is set at the red line on the tonometer holder to ensure an accurate reading.

Sometimes the assistant may find that the mires are either too thick or too thin to get a precise alignment. Thick mires indicate that too much fluorescein is present; this can be blotted from the eye and tonometer tip before remeasuring. If the mires are very thin, a little more fluorescein must be instilled in the eye before an accurate reading can be obtained. Nonoptimal mires are illustrated in Figure 9-7.

Occasionally, the assistant may misjudge the distance between the cornea and the tonometer tip, or the patient may have unnoticeably moved closer. The tonometer may be pressing too hard against the cornea once contact is made, causing the mires to appear large and widely overlapped (Figure 9-7). The instrument should be pulled slightly away from the cornea and then gently repositioned.

Applanation Pneumatonometry

The Pneumatonometer™ (Medtronics Ophthalmic, Minneapolis, Minn) employs a handheld probe with a sliding piston and pressure produced by compressed gas. The hard plastic tip has holes through which the gas passes and is covered by an elastic cap. When the flat cap applanates the anesthetized cornea, it seals the holes, creating pressure in the probe. The amount of pressure necessary to maintain the applanation is displayed on the instrument connected to the probe, as well as an estimate of the reliability of the measurement. While the central cornea is the preferred test site, this instrument has been shown to be fairly accurate in estimating the IOP when the measurement must be taken on the sclera; the measurement on the sclera tends to run 3 to 4 mm Hg higher than the corneal measurement.

Noncontact Applanation Tonometry

This instrument sends a pulse of air that flattens the cornea and then measures the time it takes to do this; it takes longer to flatten a firmer (higher IOP) cornea. The instrument rests on a table and requires the patient to be positioned in a chin rest. The measurement is taken without making contact with the eye, so the cornea does not have to be anesthetized, and the instrument can be used by less trained personnel. This method, called *air puff tonometry*, is not as accurate as

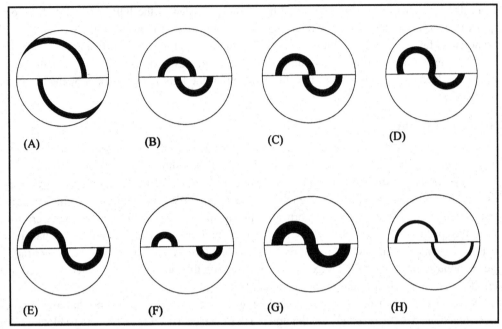

Figure 9-7. Various mires. Correct and incorrect alignment of mires. (A) Much too close. Pull slit lamp back. (B) Reading is too high. Turn knob back. (C) Correct end-point. Inner edges touch. (D) Tonometer too low. Pull back and raise it. (E) Reading is a little too low. (F) Reading is too low. Turn knob forward. (G) Too much fluorescein. (H) Not enough fluorescein. (Reprinted from Cassin B, Hamed LM, eds. *Fundamentals for Ophthalmic Personnel*. Philadelphia, Pa: WB Saunders Co; 1995.)

most other instruments, especially at higher IOPs, but is often used as a screening device. There is also a handheld version of this instrument that has a compensation feature for pressures over 30 mm Hg.

 ## Indentation Tonometry

The Schiotz tonometer was once the most widely used tonometer. It is used much less often in today's office setting, but still serves as an accurate, inexpensive, portable, autoclavable instrument for use in the operating room or in nonophthalmologic or nonoptometric settings.

The instrument is a simple mechanical device that employs a weight to press a freely moving plunger against the cornea, indenting it. The amount of indentation produced by this weight is read from a scale with a needle indicator moved by the plunger (Figure 9-8). The plunger must move freely within the cylinder of the tonometer, so the instrument must be kept scrupulously clean. Any debris or oils from the hands can accumulate in the cylinder and affect the movement of the plunger.

Cleaning the Tonometer

The entire instrument must be carefully cleaned between each patient to avoid the possible spread of infection. The instrument is made entirely of metal, so it can withstand steam sterilization and noncorrosive chemical disinfection. However, it is more common to clean the tonometer with isopropyl alcohol.

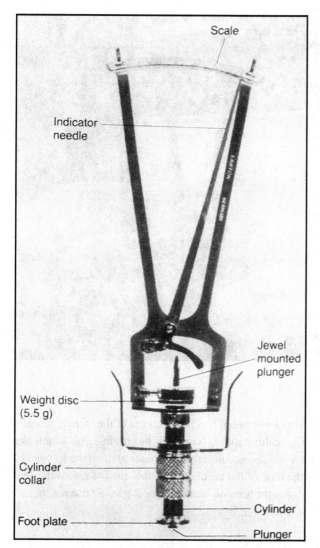

Scale

Indicator
needle

Jewel
mounted
plunger

Weight disc
(5.5 g)

Cylinder
collar

Foot plate

Cylinder

Plunger

Figure 9-8. The Schiotz tonometer. (Courtesy of Sklar Instruments.)

The instrument is disassembled by removing the weight at the top of the plunger—it snaps or screws off—and allowing the plunger to fall into the hand or onto a tissue. The cylinder is cleaned with a pipe cleaner soaked in alcohol, and the footplate is wiped clean with alcohol. The instrument is set aside to dry thoroughly because any alcohol remaining on the instrument will damage the corneal epithelium. The plunger is then cleaned with alcohol and set aside on a sterile pad to dry thoroughly. The assistant must take care not to touch the footplate or plunger with his or her bare hands once they have been cleaned. Once dry, the instrument is reassembled in reverse order, placing the notched end of the plunger into the cylinder and reattaching the weight to hold it in place. The footplate may be covered by sterile caps that are discarded after each patient. If these caps are used, the instrument does not have to be cleaned between each patient but should be cleaned at the beginning of each day.

Figure 9-9. The instrument is placed on the test block to test calibration. (Photo by Mark Arrigoni.) (Reprinted from Herrin MP. *Ophthalmic Examination and Basic Skills*. Thorofare, NJ: SLACK Incorporated; 1990.)

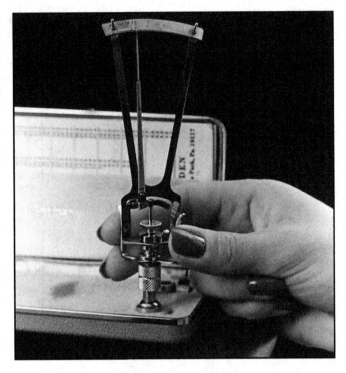

Calibrating the Schiotz

A metal test block is provided with every instrument. It is in the corner of the storage box and should be wiped clean before use. The calibration is checked by resting the tonometer perpendicularly on the test block (Figure 9-9). The needle should indicate zero on the left end of the scale. If it does not, a small screw at the base of the needle can be loosened to rezero the needle. The needle itself should be perfectly straight because bending it will give a false reading.

Performing Schiotz Tonometry

The patient must be reclining so that the eyes are looking straight up at the ceiling. A drop of anesthetic is instilled in each eye. The patient is instructed to relax and keep both eyes open and positioned straight ahead; a target placed on the ceiling is helpful. The tonometer should already have been cleaned and tested.

A right-handed assistant should hold the tonometer in the right hand using the 2 curved arms attached to the side of the cylinder. The scale mount rotates easily and should be turned so that the scale is facing the assistant. The left hand is used to gently hold the lids of the patient's right eye apart, anchoring them against the orbital rim so that no pressure is applied to the globe (Figure 9-10). An alternative hand position is to hold the upper lid with the left hand and the lower lid with the small finger of the right hand. In either case, the hand holding the tonometer can rest on the patient's cheek or forehead for stability. The tonometer is gently lowered onto the eye so that the footplate rests on the central cornea and the instrument is perpendicular. The cylinder is then lowered slightly, so that the tonometer is resting on the eye and the assistant is providing only lateral support. The cylinder should neither lift up nor press down on the footplate at this point. Looking straight at the scale, the needle position is noted. If the scale is not directly facing the assistant, an erroneous reading will be made. The tonometer is quickly lifted straight up off

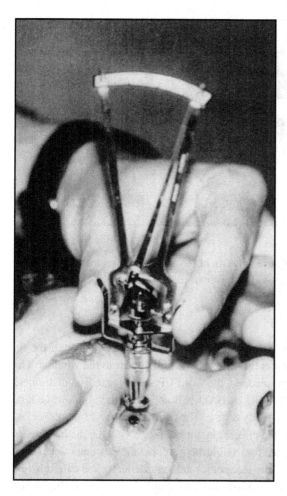

Figure 9-10. Manual technique for Schiotz tonometry. (Courtesy of Sklar Instruments.)

the cornea. Because the plunger indents the cornea, any movement of the tonometer while it is on the eye may cause an abrasion.

The scale readings do not indicate IOP in mm Hg but must be converted according to a table provided with the instrument. The scale readings are inversely proportional to the IOP; lower numbers indicate higher pressures. The standard weight on the plunger is 5.5 gm, and 2 additional weights (2.0 and 4.5 gm) may be added to this for a total of 7.5 and 10.0 gm, respectively. If the scale reading is less than 3 (ie, the IOP is more than 25), the next weight is added, and the measurement is taken again. If the 7.5 weight still gives a reading of less than 3, then the third weight is added, and the measurement is retaken. Along with the IOP, the assistant should also document the weight used.

The Tonopen™

The Tonopen is a lightweight, handheld instrument that electronically measures IOP with a modified combination of indentation and applanation. The tonometer tip has a small central disc that is pressed flush with its surrounding carrier when applied to the cornea. Pressure-sensitive electronics and a microprocessor in the handle convert the force to mm Hg and digitally display the reading and a reliability factor in a window at the top of the handle. The tonometer tip is

Figure 9-11. Technique for using the Tonopen. (Photo by Alex deLeon.)

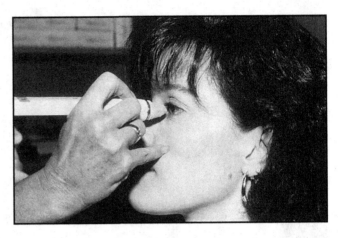

covered with a latex cap that is discarded after each patient, so no antiseptic cleaning is necessary. The instrument should always be stored with a cover in place to protect the delicate electronics from debris.

Calibrating the Instrument

The Tonopen has an internal calibration system. While holding the instrument with the tip down, the black button is quickly pressed twice; the letters CAL will appear in the window. The button is then depressed once, and after a few seconds, the word UP will appear. The instrument is then inverted so the tip is up, and either GOOD or BAD will appear in the window. GOOD indicates that the instrument is calibrated and ready to use. The calibration should be rechecked once. If BAD shows in the window and repeated checks do not produce a GOOD, the instrument cannot be used. The manual should be consulted for troubleshooting, but the instrument may have to be returned to the manufacturer for repair. The electronics are very delicate, and care must be taken not to drop or bump the instrument. A calibration check need only be done at the beginning of each day as long as the instrument has not been mishandled.

Using the Tonopen

Anesthetic is instilled in both eyes, and the patient is instructed to look straight ahead and keep both eyes open. Holding the tonometer like a pencil, with the forefinger over the black button, the instrument is directed perpendicular to the cornea (Figure 9-11). The button is pressed once to activate the instrument (a beep will be heard), and the tip is repeatedly and lightly touched to the central cornea. No pressure is applied by the assistant. A faint click is heard each time a valid reading registers. The instrument judges the reliability of each reading and then displays an average of the 4 best readings along with the overall reliability. The Tonopen is very accurate and has the advantages of portability, sterility, and reliability (even on irregular corneas). In addition, the instrument can be used in any position, so the patient can be seated, reclining, or standing.

Chapter 10

The Ocular Motility Evaluation

KEY POINTS

- Range of motion testing evaluates all 6 muscles of each eye.
- The cover/uncover test will detect the presence of a phoria or a tropia depending on which eye is being observed.
- The alternate cover (cross-cover) test does not distinguish between a phoria and a tropia.
- The alternate cover test brings out the maximum deviation.

Motility/Strabismus Screening

Eye movements are controlled by 6 muscles that are attached to each eye. The lateral rectus and medial rectus muscles move the eyes horizontally, the superior rectus and the inferior oblique muscles move the eyes up, and the inferior rectus and superior oblique muscles move the eyes down. In

addition, the vertically acting muscles also rotate the eyes to correct for a laterally tilted head position. Each muscle is innervated by 1 of 3 cranial nerves that originate in the brainstem. The individual muscles for each eye, their primary field of action, and their actions are listed in Table 10-1.

An ocular motility screening evaluation includes the range and symmetry of motion of both eyes together (versions) and each eye individually (ductions). The important gaze positions are called *cardinal positions* and are shown in Figure 10-1. While the patient holds his or her head stationary

facing the examiner, the examiner directs the patient to follow a target with the eyes only. As the patient's eyes reach each of the positions shown in Figure 10-1, the examiner evaluates whether the 2 eyes' rotation to that position has been symmetrical and whether each eye moves to the full extent of each position. If the 2 eyes' range of motion are equally full, there is no need to check the ductions. However, if one eye has failed to complete a full rotation in any direction, the opposite eye should be covered, and the weak eye should be moved to the fullest possible extent in the direction of the weakness. The weakness is recorded on a scale of 0 (no weakness/full range of motion) to -4 (maximum weakness/no movement) for each of the 6 cardinal positions of gaze. The weakness is estimated by comparison to the rotations of the normal eye.

The eyes should also be evaluated for the presence of a manifest (obvious) or latent (hidden) deviation. A manifest deviation is called a *tropia* and is observable at all times. Sometimes, a deviation is consistently observable only temporarily, such as when fusion has been broken and recovery is difficult. In this instance, the tropia is designated as *intermittent*. Tropias are categorized according to the position of the deviated (nonfixing) eye: an *inturned* eye is esotropic, an eye deviated *out* is exotropic, and when one eye is higher than the other, it is termed *hypertropic*. The classifications and their notations are listed in Table 10-2.

Tropias can be detected, classified, and measured using the corneal light reflex or the cover/uncover test. The corneal light test is performed by having the patient look at either a distant or near target while the examiner shines a penlight at the bridge of the nose. The examiner then observes whether the reflected dots of light on the patient's cornea are symmetrically positioned; normal corneal reflexes may not be centered in the pupil but may appear decentered nasally. If the corneal light reflex in one eye is shifted, a manifest deviation is present (Figure 10-2). The amount of deviation can be estimated by the Hirschberg method: 1 mm of deviation from the symmetric position is equal to about 15 prism diopters (PDs) of tropia (Figure 10-3).

The other method for determining a deviation, the cover/uncover test, is performed by having the patient fixate on either a distant or near target while the examiner covers first one eye, then the other. If the uncovered eye moves to pick up fixation (assuming at least some macular vision) when the other eye is covered, there is a tropia present. If the uncovered eye moves out, then the eye had been deviated in (esotropia); if the eye moves in, then it had been out (exotropia); if the eye moves down, then it had been up (hypertropia); and if the uncovered eye moves up, then it had been down (hypotropia). By convention, when there is a vertical deviation, it is named according to the higher eye (eg, when the right eye is down relative to the fixing left eye, the deviation is called a *left hypertropia*). If the uncovered eye does not move when the first eye is covered, the process is repeated by covering the second eye and observing the movement of the first eye. If a deviation is found, it can be measured using prisms and the cover test. This technique is covered in more detail in the Series title *A Systematic Approach to Strabismus*.

Table 10-1
Actions of the Extraocular Muscles

Muscle	Field of Action	Primary Action	Secondary Action
Medial rectus	In/nasal	Adduction (moves eye in)	
Lateral rectus	Out/temporal	Abduction (moves eye out)	
Inferior rectus	Down and out	Down in abduction	Extorsion
Superior rectus	Up and out	Up in abduction	Intorsion
Inferior oblique	Up and in	Up in adduction	Extorsion
Superior oblique	Down and in	Down in adduction	Intorsion

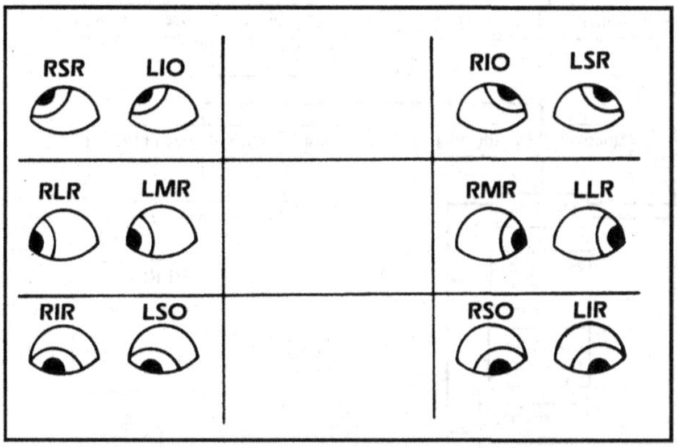

Figure 10-1. Pairs of yoke muscles responsible for moving eyes into various positions of gaze. (Reprinted from Hansen VC. *Ocular Motility*. Thorofare, NJ: SLACK Incorporated; 1986.)

Table 10-2
Classification of Common Ocular Deviations

Deviation of Eye	Classification	Notation
In	Esotropia/esophoria	ET/E
Out	Exotropia/exophoria	XT/X
Up	Hypertropia/hyperphoria	HT/H
Down	Hypotropia	hT

A phoria is a latent deviation that can only be observed when binocular fusion is disrupted. The corneal light reflex will be symmetrical. When the cover test is performed, the uncovered eye will not move to pick up fixation. However, when a phoria is present, the eye under the cover will move to re-establish fusion when the cover is removed. If the eye under the cover moves in when uncovered, the eye had been out (exophoria). Phorias usually cause no problems and generally do not have to be further evaluated. Once a phoria or a tropia has been detected, the cross-cover (or alternate cover) test may be used for measurement. The occluder is moved back and forth across the bridge of the nose to alternately cover each eye without allowing fusion. This technique elicits the largest deviation. The red glass and Maddox Rod may be used to measure phorias or tropias or to determine if there is suppression in one eye. However, since both instruments disrupt fusion, neither can distinguish between a phoria and a tropia.

Figure 10-2. The corneal light reflex of the esotropic eye is shifted temporally (at the pupillary margin). Note: The corneal reflex of the fixating eye is slightly decentered nasally. (Reprinted from Hansen VC. *Ocular Motility*. Thorofare, NJ: SLACK Incorporated; 1986.)

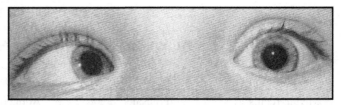

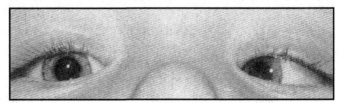

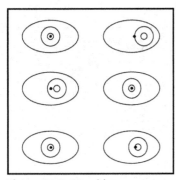

Figure 10-3. Hirschberg measurements: (Top) 90 PD left exotropia (LXT): Light reflex of the left eye deviates to the nasal limbus. (Middle) 45 PD right esotropia (RXT): Light reflex of the right eye deviates to the middle of the temporal iris. (Bottom) 30 PD LXT right reflex of the left eye deviates to the nasal pupillary border.

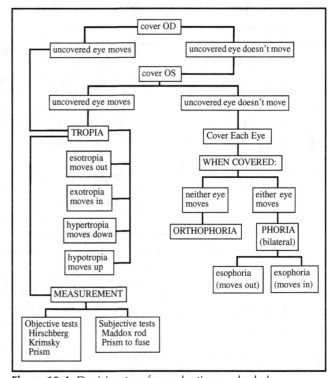

Figure 10-4. Decision tree for evaluating ocular balance.

A flow chart (Figure 10-4) demonstrates a systematic process for evaluating ocular motility

What the Patient Needs to Know

- When asked to follow a target with the eyes, do not move your head.
- During the test, keep your eyes trained on the target.

Chapter 11

Ancillary Procedures

- Stereoacuity is a binocular test and the most sensitive test of binocular function.

- Determining ocular dominance is a binocular test that may be helpful in adjusting refractive correction.

- Color vision testing is a monocular test that may help detect optic nerve or macular disorders.

- During the Schirmer tear test, lessen the patient's discomfort by dimming the lights and removing the paper strips immediately at the 5-minute mark.

- Exophthalmometry is indicated to measure ocular protrusion.

- Ophthalmic ultrasound is used as a diagnostic procedure as well as to measure the eye's internal structures.

- Check one or more vital signs to complete the new patient exam or when indicated by the patient's symptoms or interim history.

OphT

Stereoacuity

The evaluation of depth perception (stereoacuity) is the most sensitive test of binocular visual function. Fine depth perception requires good vision in both eyes, good ocular alignment, and visual fields from both eyes that overlap each other centrally. Normally, when the foveae of both eyes

OptA

are fixed on the same object in visual space, the brain melds the slightly different views from each eye (due to the separation of the eyes). The blending of these slightly different images into one produces the perception of depth.

There is a variety of informal and formal tests of depth perception. These tests are always performed with the patient using both eyes. A simple test of gross depth perception involves the patient holding the eraser end of a pencil in each hand and then touching the points to each other. A person without stereopsis will not be able to move the pencils so that the points are touching (Figure 11-1). More formal tests of stereopsis allow quantification of the results. Stereopsis is measured in seconds (sec) of arc, with a smaller number indicating better or finer stereopsis.

Formal tests of stereoacuity typically utilize Polaroid glasses that allow each eye to view displaced images that have been specially printed in a test booklet (Figure 11-2). If a patient has only very coarse stereoacuity, he or she may only be able to perceive the fly on a Wirt test as being 3-dimensional; this corresponds to 3000 sec of arc. If the patient has fine stereoacuity, he or she will be able to appreciate all of the animals and most of the circles on a Wirt test as 3-dimensional. The last test diamond represents the finest stereoacuity, and when the correct circle is identified, it means the patient has at least 40 sec of arc stereoacuity. The seconds of arc for each test section are listed in the literature that accompanies the test. The last figure (circle or animal) correctly identified is the measure of a patient's level of stereoacuity and can be documented according to the test pamphlet. If the pamphlet is not available, the level can be documented as the number of correct responses in each section (eg, 6/9 circles [6 correct out of 9 possible]). Other similar tests employ figures such as triangles and stars that are placed in different areas of a uniform background and can only be seen with dissociating glasses.

Because these are tests of binocular function, it is important that nothing has been done prior to the test that might possibly interfere with fusion. Glasses should not be removed, neither eye should be occluded, and the patient should be allowed to use an abnormal head position if this permits the best possible binocular function. Anyone, child or adult, who uses bifocals should be instructed to use the near segment (with the polarizing glasses over them) while performing these tests.

What the Patient Needs to Know

- For the depth perception test, put the dark glasses over your own glasses and look through your bifocals (or use your reading glasses).

- Hold the test booklet about 14 in away, and make sure you have good light.

CL

Ocular Dominance

Occasionally, it is useful to know which of the patient's eyes is dominant. The dominant eye is unconsciously used for sighting distant objects or viewing with a monocular eyepiece and is not necessarily the same as a person's hand dominance. Determining ocular dominance is especially important when fitting contact lenses for monovision (usually the dominant eye for distance and the other for near). Ocular dominance in an adult may be easily determined by having the patient make

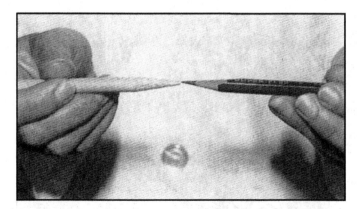

Figure 11-1. Pencil point to pencil point test for gross stereopsis. (Top) Patient with stereopsis is able to touch points. (Bottom) Patient without stereopsis cannot touch points. (Reprinted from Hansen VC. *Ocular Motility*. Thorofare, NJ: SLACK Incorporated; 1986.)

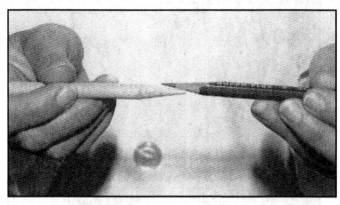

a small triangle with his or her hands, overlapping the forefingers and thumbs and keeping the other fingers together. With the hand triangle resting in his or her lap, the patient is instructed to sight a small object (such as a light switch or door lock) on a distant wall straight ahead *with both eyes open*. Then, the patient is instructed to raise the triangle straight up from the lap to center the distant object in the triangle while continuing to look at the object with both eyes (Figure 11-3). With the object still centered, the patient can determine which eye was used to sight and center the object by closing first one eye and then the other. This should be repeated once or twice for verification. When the patient is a young child, he or she can point to the object and then the examiner alternately covers the patient's eyes. The nondominant eye will require a hand shift to resight the object. Other methods of determining ocular dominance, such as asking the patient which eye is used for aiming, are described in the BSS Contact Lens book.

What the Patient Needs to Know

- For the ocular dominance test, keep both eyes open and raise your hands directly in front of you to sight the target.

- You will be asked to first close one eye then the other to determine which eye sighted the target. Do not move your hands during this part of the test.

Figure 11-2. Testing stereopsis. (Photo by Mark Arrigoni.) (Reprinted from Herrin MP. *Ophthalmic Examination and Basic Skills*. Thorofare, NJ: SLACK Incorporated; 1990.)

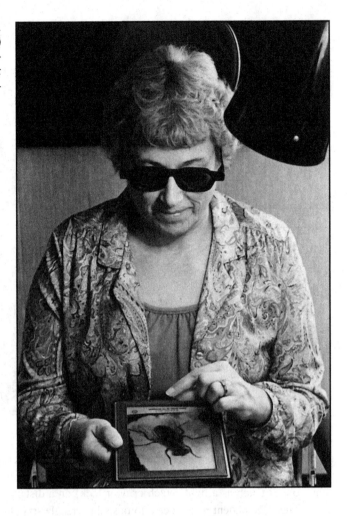

Color Vision Plates

Color vision defects may be hereditary or acquired. Most hereditary defects are transmitted by the mother and usually affect male offspring; hereditary color blindness occurs in 8% to 10% of males and in less than 0.5% of females. Because the defective gene is recessive, many more females carry the gene than actually have a color vision defect. Acquired color blindness occurs when the macular photoreceptors, the cones, have been damaged by optic nerve or macular disorders.

The cones have 3 different pigments that process visible light as red, green, blue, or some mixture of these. There may be partial or complete loss of one or more of these pigments. When there is a red defect, this color appears less intense, so colors that have red in their mixture may be confused with other colors. The most common color vision defect is red-green confusion. Complete color blindness is rare and is associated with poor vision and nystagmus; all colors are perceived as shades of gray. Fortunately, the most common defects of color vision are not severe, and visual acuity is unaffected.

There are a variety of tests to assess color vision. Some of the early tests required the patient to match colored yarns or colored glass panes in a lantern. Modern tests range from identification of figures on test plates (Ishihara or Hardy-Rand-Rittler) to the more time-consuming

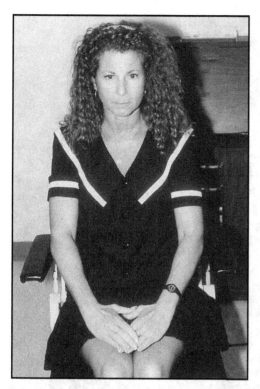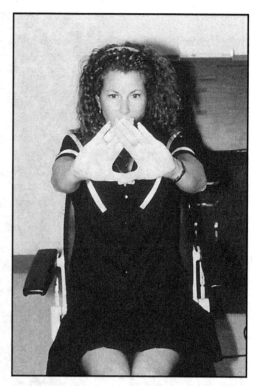

Figure 11-3. Determining ocular dominance. (A) The patient forms a small triangle with the hands resting in the lap while viewing a distant object with both eyes. (B) With both eyes open, the triangle is raised straight up and the object is sighted through it. The patient then determines which eye can see the object in the triangle. (Photo by Alex deLeon.)

arrangement of colored caps in a tray (D-15 or FM-100 tests, discussed in detail in the Series title *Special Skills and Techniques*).

The color vision test most often used in the office is the Ishihara Pseudoisochromatic plates. These plates have colored dots that form numbers against a dotted background of another color (Figure 11-4). The patient views the plates under good illumination separately with each eye. The first plate in the booklet is a test plate that is easy to distinguish and intended to show the patient how the test works. A person with normal color vision will be able to identify most of the remaining numbers; 1 or 2 of the plates are difficult for most people and do not distinguish between normal and abnormal color vision. A color deficient person will either misidentify certain numbers or not see them at all. This test will show complete color blindness or red-green confusion but does not quantify color deficiencies. The results of this test are documented by noting the number of color plates correctly identified out of the number of possible correct answers. There are some plates that do not have test numbers, but rather a colored line that winds through a different colored background. These plates are for young or illiterate patients and are used by having the patient trace the colored line.

The Ishihara test is also useful in following patients recovering from temporary optic nerve disorders (such as optic neuritis) who regain at least some of their color vision.

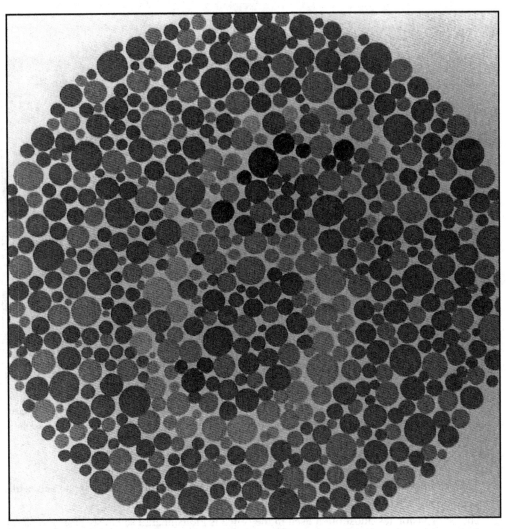

Figure 11-4. Black and white photo of a multi-hue 6 within a circle of random dots of opposite hues. (Reprinted from Benes SC, McKinney K, Sanders LC, Herrin M, Moberg M. *Advanced Ophthalmic Diagnostics and Therapeutics*. Thorofare, NJ: SLACK Incorporated; 1992.)

What the Patient Needs to Know

- The color vision plates may seem confusing, but look for 1 or 2 large numerals in the colored circles.

- The test is performed on each eye separately, and your reading glasses or bifocals may be used.

Schirmer Tear Test

Many of the complaints we hear, especially from older patients, are of a somewhat vague ocular discomfort that may be the result of a deficiency in tear production or composition. A defect in any

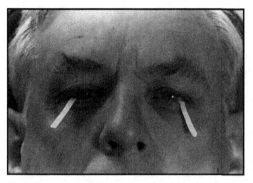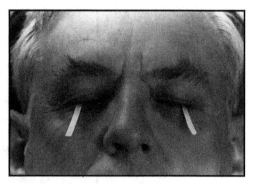

Figure 11-5. Schirmer test. (Photo by Mark Arrig ni.) (Reprinted from Herrin MP. *Ophthalmic Examination and Basic Skills*. Thorofare, NJ: SLACK Incorporated; 1990.)

1 of the 3 components of the tear film (mucin, aqueous, or lipid) may contribute to insufficient or inefficient corneal lubrication and protection. Paradoxically, some patients with a dry eye sometimes notice excessive tearing, but this is the lacrimal gland's normal response to corneal surface irritation; these reflex tears are not of sufficient quality to solve the problem.

The Schirmer test is the most convenient way to assess tear deficiency in the office setting. In Schirmer's Test I, one end of a sterile standardized filter paper strip is inserted a few millimeters under the lower lid just temporal to the cornea (Figure 11-5). The eye is not anesthetized, so the irritation caused by the paper strip causes reflex tearing. The patient is instructed to keep the eyes gently closed for 5 minutes. The strip is then carefully removed, and the length of the strip that has become moistened with tears is measured. A normal eye should produce enough tears to wet at least 10 mm of the strip in 5 minutes. Older patients may have slightly less wetting. When significantly less wetting is measured, the patient is considered to have a dry eye and may be treated with ocular lubricants (artificial tears, ointments), punctum occlusion (either temporary or permanent), or both. This test may also be used when evaluating a prospective contact lens wearer.

Another tear test, Schirmer's Test II, is performed using a topical anesthetic to avoid the tearing caused by the paper strip irritating the eye. This test measures baseline tear function and usually shows less paper strip wetting.

What the Patient Needs to Know

- The tear test may be a little uncomfortable, but keep your eyes gently closed, and relax.

- The strips will be removed in just 5 minutes.

Exophthalmometry

`OphA`

Abnormal protrusion of one or both eyes is called *proptosis* (or *exophthalmos*). Proptosis is caused by an increased mass in the orbit behind the globe. Because the bony orbit is rigid, any increase in the volume of its contents will push the globe forward.

The most common cause of increased mass in the orbit is Graves disease. In this thyroid-related disorder, the extraocular muscles and other orbital tissues are infiltrated with inflammatory fibrotic material and become both enlarged and inelastic. This process not only pushes the globe forward but

Figure 11-6. Exophthalmometer. (Courtesy of Bausch and Lomb.) (Reprinted from Herrin MP. *Ophthalmic Examination and Basic Skills*. Thorofare, NJ: SLACK Incorporated; 1990.)

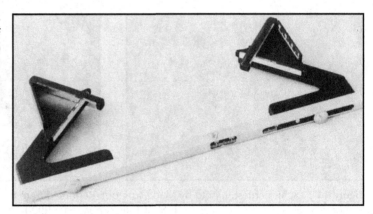

also limits its movement because the orbital tissues are engorged and stiff. The muscles of the eyelids are also involved; the levator cannot relax and the upper lid retracts. This lid retraction exposes more of the eyeball, making the proptosis seem more severe and making the eye itself seem larger. Other disorders that might have a similar effect in the posterior orbit are space-occupying lesions such as tumors, cysts, and hematomas, or inflammatory processes, such as orbital cellulitis.

Sometimes one eye may seem to protrude, but it only appears that way because the other eye is abnormally recessed in the orbit. Backward displacement of the globe is called *enophthalmos* and may occur if there is loss of orbital mass, as with degeneration of muscle or orbital fat. Enophthalmos will make the globe seem small because the lid will rest at a lower position on the front of the eye.

It is important to measure the position of the globes in their orbits if there is apparent exophthalmos, enophthalmos, or asymmetry. The globe is usually positioned at the front of the orbit so that in primary gaze, the anterior point of the cornea is 12 to 20 mm in front of the plane of the orbital opening. The average distance between the lateral orbit rim and the corneal apex is 16 to 18 mm; there should be no more than 1 to 2 mm difference between the measurements of the 2 eyes.

The Hertel exophthalmometer is a handheld instrument that uses mirrors to help the examiner visualize the eye from the side and measure the position of the corneal apex with respect to the lateral orbital rim (Figure 11-6). The examiner holds the instrument in both hands with the mirrored triangles toward the patient. The metal notches at the back of the mirror housings are placed firmly against both lateral orbits at the lateral canthi but not touching the globe (Figure 11-7). Correct placement of the instrument might be slightly uncomfortable for the patient, but the examiner should not push so hard as to cause pain. The numbers on the front of the bar represent the distance between the right and left lateral orbital rims. This measurement is recorded in millimeters as the BASE. For future measurements, the instrument will be set at the same base number to allow for serial comparisons of the eye position.

With the patient looking straight ahead and the exophthalmometer held parallel to the floor, the examiner shifts slightly to the left and aligns the red lines visible in the left mirror. Keeping the red lines aligned, the examiner then notes the position of the right eye's corneal apex on the millimeter rule in the mirror. The left eye position is measured in the same manner by the examiner's shifting *slightly* to the right. The numbers for each eye are recorded along with the base number. Because the notches make contact with the patient, they should be wiped with alcohol between each patient.

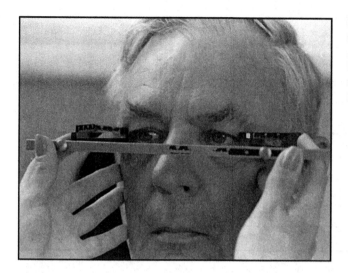

Figure 11-7. Measuring exophthalmos on a patient. (Photo by Mark Arrigoni.) (Reprinted from Herrin MP. *Ophthalmic Examination and Basic Skills.* Thorofare, NJ: SLACK Incorporated; 1990.)

A less accurate method of measurement is to simply hold a millimeter rule against each lateral rim and measure the distance to the corneal apex. With this method, there will be no base measurement, and the possibility for error will be greater.

Sometimes, it is difficult to tell whether one eye is exophthalmic or the other is enophthalmic. The patient's history and other diagnostic tests usually settle the question, but accurate sequential measurements may contribute significantly to making the correct diagnosis.

What the Patient Needs to Know

- This test is to measure any protrusion of your eye(s).

- You should be seated comfortably and remove your glasses.

- The instrument will be placed against your outer eye sockets and may be slightly uncomfortable, but not painful.

- Keep both eyes open and look straight ahead while the examiner moves from side to side.

A-Scan Biometry

OphA

Just as properties of light allow us to see structures in the eye, sound may be used to evaluate the tissue through which it passes. Sound has many of the same characteristics of light, such as reflection and absorption, and special instruments have been developed to use ultrasound (which is not audible) as a diagnostic tool. The velocity of sound changes as it travels through different tissues, and this information is captured by the instrument and presented in numeric and graphic forms.

The ultrasound instrument probe emits the sound waves. The sound waves change speed as they travel through the eye and encounter different types of tissue. At the interface between tissue types (eg, aqueous/lens or vitreous/retina), sound is either transmitted or reflected. The sound waves that are reflected return to the probe where they are detected, amplified, and then displayed on a small screen on the instrument. The display shows a series of spikes corresponding to the tissue interfaces.

Figure 11-8. A-scan tracing showing high, steeply rising spikes and baseline millimeter scale. (Courtesy of Rhonda G. Waldron, Eye Scan Consulting.)

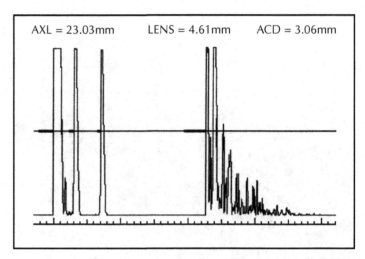

AXL = 23.03mm   LENS = 4.61mm   ACD = 3.06mm

The greater the reflected signal from an interface, the higher the spike will be. Since the spikes represent the anterior and posterior surfaces of ocular structures, their relative locations in the eye are easily demonstrated, and measurements can be made from the millimeter scale along the bottom of the tracing (Figure 11-8). This technique is known as *ocular echography* (the recording of echoes).

The most commonly performed type of ocular echography is the A-scan. The A stands for *amplitude* and refers to amplification or height of the echoes, a measure of the time it takes for the emitted sound waves to return to the probe. The term *biometry* refers to the measurement of the structures and spaces in the eye. This type of scan provides a 1-dimensional readout.

Another use of ophthalmic ultrasound, the B-scan, is more diagnostic; echoes are displayed as a cross sectional picture of the eye. Intraocular abnormalities that are not visible due to media problems (such as cataract) may be detected with B-scan, which gives a 2-dimensional view in real time. A description of this type of ultrasound may be found in the Series text, *Special Skills and Techniques*.

The biometric evaluation of the eye using A-scan allows monitoring of ocular diseases such as congenital glaucoma, in which the young eye grows abnormally large (buphthalmos), or of intraocular or orbital tumors, whereby the dimensions of the mass can be tracked. The most common use of A-scan biometry, however, is to determine the axial length of the eye as well as the size of the structures and compartments within the eye. The axial measurement can help diagnose microphthalmia (small eye) or determine whether an abnormally long eye is contributing to high myopia. A-scan measurements are probably most often used in the calculations to determine the power of the IOL that is implanted to replace the natural lens when a cataract is surgically removed (see *IOL Calculations* on next page).

The best quality echo spikes (highest and most perpendicular to the baseline) are produced when the sound waves strike the surface of a structure perpendicular to the plane of that surface (Figure 11-9). This maximizes the echo and allows for more exact measurement of the distances between echo spikes. The distance between spikes depends on the time it takes for the sound to travel from surface to surface. Knowing the velocity of sound through various intraocular structures permits the calculation of the distance between them as well as the total distance from the front of the eye to the back (axial length). The velocity of sound through ocular tissues or materials is listed in Table 11-1.

Figure 11-9. Echoes striking perpendicular to the ocular surface (A) produce the highest spikes and most accurate measurements compared with nonperpendicular echoes (B,C). (Courtesy of Rhonda G. Waldron, Eye Scan Consulting.)

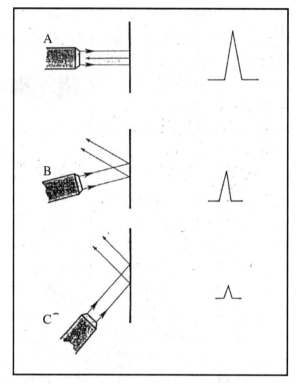

Table 11-1

Ocular Tissues/Materials	Velocity of Sound
Normal cornea and lens	1641 m/sec
Average cataract	1550 m/sec
Aqueous and vitreous	1532 m/sec
Silicone IOL	1486 m/sec
PMMA IOL	2718 m/sec
Acrylic IOL	2120 m/sec
Silicone oil	980 m/sec

Higher velocity (faster) waves do not penetrate tissue or material as well as lower velocity waves, so the faster waves echo back to the probe producing a higher spike. Echoes that produce the highest and most perpendicular spikes are those that strike interfaces directly and not at an angle. The most accurate intraocular measurements come from scans in which the sound waves travel precisely along the visual axis (central cornea to fovea). The ultrasonographer must determine and capture the highest quality scan during the testing (next section).

Procedure

There are 2 methods for performing A-scan biometry: applanation (contact) and immersion (noncontact). Applanation is probably more widely used, as it is easy, quick, and is performed with the patient sitting up. It has the same disadvantages of other procedures that touch the cornea, such as the possibility of infection transmission and errors related to compression of the cornea.

Figure 11-10. Applanation (Contact) A-scan tracing showing 5 equally high spikes. (Illustration by M. Bryan Waldron.) (Courtesy of Rhonda G. Waldron, Eye Scan Consulting.)

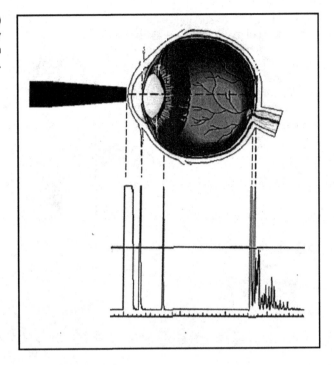

Immersion biometry does not require that the probe touch the eye, so infection and corneal compression are not an issue. However, the patient must be lying down, and the method uses a fluid- or gel-filled reservoir on the eye, which requires more time and can be messy.

Prior to beginning the measurement with either method, the instrument must be set for phakic (natural lens, cataract), pseudophakic (IOL), or aphakic (no lens) calculations, depending on the status of the eye being measured. Check the operator's manual for specific instructions regarding setting gate positions (spaces to be measured), gain adjustments (amount of amplification of echoes), etc.

Applanation (Contact) Biometry

The patient is seated comfortably at the chin rest and the instrument is placed so the operator can easily see the screen while performing the test. The procedure is much like applanation tonometry. After explaining the procedure to the patient, the operator anesthetizes the eyes with a topical drop (eg, proparacaine), and the patient is instructed to look straight ahead and keep the eyes still. Maintaining an adequate tear film is important for good sound wave transmission, so the patient must be allowed to blink between measurements, and each measurement should be as brief as possible (<10 sec). The probe is positioned at the center of the cornea and perpendicular to the anterior plane of the cornea. The probe is moved toward the cornea until contact is made (ie, spikes are seen on the instrument screen). The probe may be slightly adjusted vertically and/or horizontally to achieve the best alignment and, therefore, the optimum spike configuration. Five spikes are seen: the cornea, the anterior and posterior lens surfaces, the retina, and the sclera. In the normal eye, all spikes should be equally high and sharply rising (Figure 11-10).

Some probes are handheld, which allows the operator more flexibility in alignment. Some instruments automatically freeze "acceptable" scans, but the parameters are programmed into the instrument by the manufacturer and may not accurately reflect the conditions of the particular measurement. The operator may elect to use a foot pedal to choose appropriate scans.

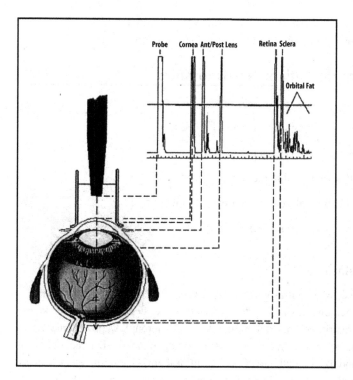

Figure 11-11. Immersion (noncontact) A-scan tracing showing 6 high spikes. (Illustration by M. Bryan Waldron.) (Courtesy of Rhonda G. Waldron, Eye Scan Consulting.)

What the Patient Needs to Know

- This test is to measure the structures inside your eye.

- Be sure you are seated comfortably and breathing normally.

- Keep both eyes open with the lids relaxed (not squeezing).

- Do not move your head or eyes during the test.

- You will be given an opportunity to blink between measurements.

Immersion (Noncontact) Biometry

Immersion biometry is performed using a tubular scleral shell that is filled with saline or methylcellulose to provide the initial medium for the sound waves. The patient must be lying down when the shell is positioned and filled, and care must be taken that there are no bubbles present in the fluid. Some shells are a closed system once the probe is inserted, which then allows the patient to sit up for the actual measurement. The probe is immersed in the fluid to a depth near the apex of the cornea but not touching it.

Immersion biometry yields 6 spikes, the first 2 of which are actually double-peaked and represent the corneal epithelium and endothelium. The final 4 spikes represent the same structures as the applanation method. (Figure 11-11) Immersion is the more accurate method for measuring axial length because the probe cannot indent the cornea and thereby artificially shorten the eye. Just as the applanation instrument either automatically freezes certain scans or responds to a foot pedal, the immersion instrument also has both automated and manual modes. It is best to use the manual mode so that the operator can decide on the quality of the scans and which to freeze. Since the scans may be averaged to arrive at the axial length measurement, it is important to evaluate each captured scan and immediately delete any that have low spikes and/or spikes that are not perpendicular.

What the Patient Needs to Know

- This test is to measure the structures inside your eye.

- You will be sitting up (or reclining if immersion) for this test.

- Breathe normally and keep both eyes open.

- Do not move your head or eyes during the test.

- A small fluid-filled cup will be placed on your eye (if immersion).

- Let the technician know if you become anxious or uncomfortable.

Intraocular Lens Calculations

IOL powers may be calculated by the ultrasound instrument itself or by using a computer program in which the A-scan measurements (axial length, anterior chamber depth, and lens thickness) and keratometer measurements are primarily used for computation. Different IOL power calculation formulas use other biometric data, such as refractive error and corneal diameter, but accurate measurements of corneal curvature and axial length are critical to all of them. One millimeter of difference in the axial length corresponds to about 3 D of change in the refractive error of the eye, so a small error in measurement can have a large effect on the postoperative refractive error (AKA, "the post-op surprise").

Vital Signs

Occasionally, it is necessary for the eyecare professional to monitor a patient's vital signs in the office. This includes measuring blood pressure using a pressure cuff (sphygmomanometer) and stethoscope, taking the pulse (heart rate), counting respirations (breathing rate), and taking the temperature.

Blood Pressure

The pressure cuff is firmly secured, but not tight, around the patient's upper arm. If the patient has exerted him- or herself getting into the room or chair, blood pressure should not be measured for a few minutes. All clothing sleeves should be positioned loosely above the cuff, and the pressure gauge should be positioned so that its face is clearly visible to the examiner. The patient should have his or her arm extended, palm up, so that the flat surface of the stethoscope membrane can be held firmly against the inner elbow. The bulb attached to the cuff is used to force air into the cuff; the bulb has a metal screw valve that opens and closes this airway.

The patient is instructed to breathe normally and remain still throughout the procedure. With the stethoscope earpieces in place, the stethoscope membrane against the patient's inner elbow, the cuff gauge visible, and the bulb valve in the closed position (ie, air can be pumped into but cannot escape the cuff), the examiner begins to pump air into the cuff by repeatedly squeezing the bulb (Figure 11-12). At a point usually between 80 and 110 mm Hg on the gauge, the heartbeat will become audible to the examiner. Enough air must be pumped into the cuff so that

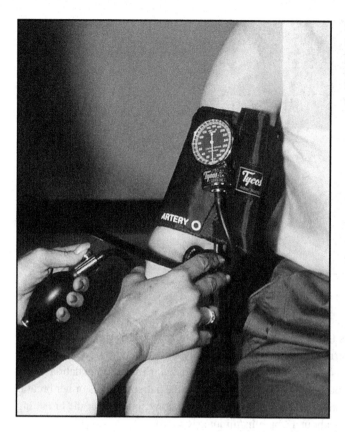

Figure 11-12. The blood pressure cuff is adjusted so that the pressure gauge is clearly visible. The stethoscope membrane is placed against the inner elbow. (Photo by Alex deLeon.)

this sound is no longer heard. At this point, the bulb valve is barely opened to allow the air in the cuff to escape slowly. The examiner, listening carefully, notes the number on the gauge at which the heartbeat first becomes audible again; this is the *systolic* pressure and is usually 110 to 140 mm Hg. The examiner continues to slowly let air out of the cuff and notes the gauge reading at which the heartbeat sound again disappears; this is the *diastolic* pressure (normally 70 to 90 mm Hg). The blood pressure is recorded with the higher number (systolic pressure) over the lower number (diastolic pressure), as in 134/86. Documentation should include which arm was used and the patient's position (sitting, reclining, etc) during the test.

Heart Rate

The pulse (heart rate) is taken using a clock or watch with a second hand. The examiner places his or her first 2 fingers—never the thumb—over the lateral aspect of the patient's inner wrist when the palm is turned up (Figure 11-13). The heartbeat can be felt in the groove between the outer wristbone and the central cords. The examiner need not apply much pressure to the wrist to be able to feel the pulse. Once the pulse is identified, the number of beats in a minute is counted. The experienced examiner may elect to count for 30 seconds and multiply the number of beats by 2 to get the heart rate. If the pulse cannot be felt at the wrist, the examiner may use the neck pulse in the depression on either side of the windpipe. However, the examiner must use the lightest possible touch, because this is a large blood vessel that supplies the brain. The normal adult heart rate is about 72 beats/minute (HR = 72).

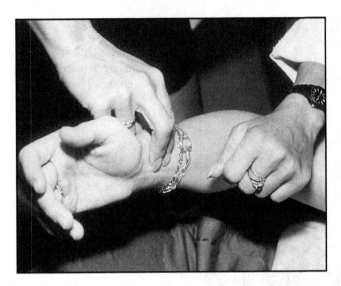

Figure 11-13. Find the pulse at the lateral aspect of the upturned wrist. (Photo by Alex deLeon.)

Respirations

It is easy to count the breaths taken in a minute by continuing to watch the clock's second hand after the pulse has been determined. The examiner merely shifts his or her attention to the rise and fall of the patient's chest as each breath is taken and exhaled. Either the inhalation or the exhalation should be counted, not both. By not expressly alerting the patient that his or her breathing is now being monitored, the patient will not be triggered to unconsciously alter the breathing pattern. Normal adult respiration is about 18 breaths/minute (R = 18).

Temperature

Body temperature is generally taken with a glass thermometer that contains a thin column of gray mercury (Hg) or a red liquid. The thermometer is cleaned with a disinfectant solution between patients. When ready for use, the assistant should grasp the clear end of the thermometer firmly and shake the mercury down into the reservoir; the thin column should be very short at this point. The liquid reservoir end of the thermometer is placed under the patient's tongue and allowed to remain there with the mouth closed until the column has reached its maximum height (usually in 3 or 4 min). The top of the column is read against a scale printed on the glass. If the reading is not at least 98° F, the thermometer should be repositioned under the patient's tongue for another minute or 2 to make sure the temperature is accurate. The normal temperature is about 98.6°F. Newer thermometers use a temperature sensor that is placed under the tongue or in the outer ear canal and give a digital readout.

What the Patient Needs to Know

- It is important to breathe normally, be relaxed and quiet, and sit still in order to get accurate blood pressure and pulse readings.

- When your temperature is being taken, keep the thermometer under your tongue, do not bite down, keep your mouth closed, and breathe through your nose.

Chapter 12

Assisting in Minor Surgery

KEY POINTS

- You must be meticulous about microbial control and sterility in the surgical arena.

- Be cognizant of sources of contamination.

- Be sensitive to the patient's apprehension.

- Discretion and protection of the patient's privacy are very important in the surgical setting.

- Assume only as much responsibility as the physician allows.

- Make the physician aware of any patient problems that arise before, during, or after surgery.

- Familiarize yourself with the operation of any instrument for which you will have responsibility.

The eyecare professional, working in concert with the physician and other clinical or surgical personnel, is responsible for maintaining a clean and/or sterile environment suitable for minor surgical procedures. This requires strict adherence to accepted standards of microbial control including sterilization of instruments, use of sterile technique, preparation of the surgical site, and control of the surgical environment. In addition, surgical personnel are often called upon to assist the surgeon by handling certain equipment (lasers, cautery, etc) or by directly participating in the procedure itself. The surgeon depends on the surgical staff for the organization and efficiency that contribute to a safe, calm experience for the patient. Minor procedures are usually performed in a special room in the clinic, in an examination room, or in an outpatient facility affiliated with the clinic. Assisting in major ocular surgery is covered in the Series title *The Ophthalmic Surgical Assistant.*

Microbial Control

Universal precautions is a term that cautions the health care worker to treat every patient as if he or she has an infectious disease. Hand washing is perhaps the single most effective barrier to the transmission of infectious agents (microbes), such as bacteria or viruses. It is reassuring to the patient if the eyecare professional washes his or her hands in the presence of the patient prior to the examination or procedure. Of course, the hands must also be washed after contact with each patient. The same is true of keeping clinic equipment clean. When the patient sees clean surfaces and watches the cleaning of chin rests, forehead bands, and tonometer tips, he or she will be assured of the assistant's attention to patient safety.

In the minor surgery setting, the assistant is in charge of keeping the room well stocked and scrupulously clean. In addition, the assistant is responsible for cleaning and sterilizing surgical instruments and supplies. Most items are amenable to pressurized steam sterilization (autoclave), which is the most common, convenient, and effective method of sterilization. Some items, such as powders or instruments with glued or cemented parts, require dry, chemical, or gas sterilization. Consult product labels and owners' manuals for proper sterilization of such objects.

All instruments must be clean and free of organic debris (blood, tissue, etc) before being placed in the autoclave. Hinged instruments, such as forceps or scissors, should be open when placed in the autoclave, and spaced so that the steam can contact as much of each instrument's surface as possible. When instruments are to be sterilized and then stored, each item is wrapped in cloth or paper or placed in a paper envelope. These packages are sealed with sensitized tape that indicates when sterilization has taken place. The tape must be marked with the date of sterilization and the initials of the assistant. An unopened sterilized package can be stored for up to 30 days before it must be rewrapped and resterilized.

Proper disposal of contaminated items greatly reduces the possibility of microbe transmission. Items soiled with tissue or body fluids should be deposited in a sealable plastic bag and marked for careful handling and/or disposal. Sharp items (called *sharps*) such as needles or blades are always placed in a rigid red plastic container that is sealed when it is full. This container will be delivered to or picked up by a company that will properly dispose of it. Sharps should be dropped into the container point first, and one should never reach into the container. Neither blades nor needles should be resheathed before disposal because this practice increases the chance of sticking one's self. If the assistant's skin is penetrated by a used blade or needle, *it must be reported immediately.* Every effort must be made to avoid the possibility of transmitting any microbes, especially those causing AIDS and hepatitis.

Aseptic Technique

Aseptic technique is a method of microbial control that promotes sterile conditions and the maximum possible cleanliness in a surgical area. All personnel in the surgical area must understand and adhere to the rules governing aseptic technique. Sources of contamination are everywhere in the operating room, including airborne dust, dirt on the floor, dirty furniture surfaces, unsterile supplies, and especially the people who enter the room (surgeon, assistants, and the patient).

The main principle of aseptic technique is that only sterile surfaces may touch each other and only unsterile surfaces may touch each other. If the assistant is wearing sterile gloves, then the gloved hands may only touch other sterile items. Any sterile item that touches something nonsterile is then considered contaminated and must be removed from the sterile area; it may not be used again in the sterile field. If a gloved hand becomes contaminated, the glove must be changed.

The patient's face may be covered with a sterile drape or merely prepped with disinfectants. In either case, the patient should be cautioned not to touch his or her face and then monitored for reflexive scratching or touching of the prepped area. The assistant must constantly be aware of sources of contamination and alert the appropriate person if a breach of sterility has been noticed.

Because the minor procedure room is equipped to handle less invasive types of surgical procedures, only local anesthetics (topical or injected) are used. Often, only one person will assist the surgeon in these cases. This assistant may be responsible for setting up the instrument tray and any equipment to be used, positioning and prepping the patient, retrieving items requested during the procedure, assisting with the procedure itself, medicating and patching the operated eye, processing the appropriate paperwork, and cleaning the room and instruments afterward. This means the assistant must always be cognizant of what is sterile because he or she will be shifting in and out of being sterile and being able to touch those items.

Although minor procedures do not usually require personnel to wear caps, masks, and shoe covers, there are a few things the assistant can do to help minimize contamination. Fingernails should be kept short, neat, and clean; frequent hand washing during the day is imperative. If hair is longer than shoulder length, it should be held back with a clip or band. A separate pair of working shoes can be kept in the office so that street shoes are kept out of the procedure room. An alternative is to have carpeting or a mat outside the room for wiping the feet. Finally, it is best not to bring a known infection, such as a cold or open wound, into the procedure room.

The best preventive measure is constant awareness of the sterile environment and one's place in it.

Minor Surgery Procedures

Minor procedures are generally limited to the lids and external eye and require only local anesthesia and a reassured patient. A brief description of common procedures follows.

Lids

Some procedures may be done in the exam room or at the slit lamp. These include, but are not limited to, removal of lashes (epilation), suture removal, or adjustment of sutures.

In addition to prepping the patient and the surgical area, the assistant may also assist the surgeon directly by keeping the incision site clean, cutting sutures, loading needleholders, etc.

Lesions

Small benign lesions such as skin tags or papillomae are easily excised from the skin and may not require sutures. Other lesions, such as basal cell carcinomas (BCC), even if very small, require deeper excisions to prevent the spread of the cancer. If the BCC is large, lid reconstruction may be warranted at the time of the procedure.

A chalazion is a common intralid lesion that has not resolved with medical therapy. In these cases, the lid is inverted, and the chalazion is incised so that its inflammatory contents can be removed. This incision is self-sealing and requires no sutures.

Blepharoplasty

This procedure removes excess skin and anterior orbital fat from the upper and/or lower lids. Because this involves a full-thickness excision of the lid skin, control of bleeding and prevention of infection is very important. Anesthesia is accomplished by subcutaneous injection of a local anesthetic such as lidocaine. Epinephrine may be injected along with the anesthetic to prolong anesthesia and help control bleeding.

Lacrimal Probe/Irrigation

Occasionally, the lacrimal drainage system has failed to open at birth or has become closed due to inflammation or trauma. In these cases, special instruments are used to probe and gently open the channel either mechanically or by irrigation.

External Eye

Refractive Surgery

There are several popular methods for surgically correcting myopia (nearsightedness), and new methods are being developed. Myopia results when the corneal curvature is steep enough to focus light rays in front of the retina or when the eye is too long for the focus of a flatter cornea. In either event, changing (flattening) the corneal curvature will move the focal point closer to the retina, producing clearer distance vision. This elective procedure has become so common that entire surgical centers are dedicated to doing this type of surgery.

The primary method used before the early 1990s was radial keratotomy (RK). This procedure involves making 4 or 8 radial incisions in the cornea from the limbus to about 3 mm from the center of the cornea and extending through about 95% of the cornea's thickness. This causes a flattening of the cornea (decreasing its curvature) and lessens the myopia. This procedure requires only topical anesthetic drops and 3 or 4 instruments, takes only a few minutes to perform, and is relatively painless.

Another type of incisional refractive surgery is astigmatic keratotomy (AK). Astigmatism occurs when different meridians of the cornea have different curvatures. AK employs circumferential rather than radial incisions. The principle of flattening corneal curvature is the same. A corneal incision made parallel to the limbus at the steepest meridian will lessen the amount of astigmatism.

The excimer laser became increasingly popular in refractive surgery. It was first approved in the mid-1990s to obliterate superficial corneal scars and to smooth irregular corneal surfaces. It was more recently approved to perform keratectomy for myopia (PRK). The laser removes a flat disc of corneal tissue by destroying cells (ablation) in Bowman's layer. When the procedure is for the correction of myopia, sequential thin layers of tissue are destroyed until a level is reached (predetermined by the laser's computer) to correct a given amount of myopia. This procedure also requires only topical anesthetic. In preparation for the laser procedure, the epithelial layer is removed, and during the 3 or 4 days it takes for the epithelium to regenerate, the patient may experience mild to severe pain (loss of the epithelium is a huge corneal abrasion). Also, the laser sometimes produces a haze in Bowman's layer. Most patients are not bothered by this, but it may be severe enough to interfere with vision. It may be several weeks before the patient can appreciate the best vision produced by the laser procedure.

Modifications of the excimer laser procedure for myopia have been designed to avoid postoperative haze. This new procedure does not require the removal of the epithelium. Instead, it involves cutting a small, partially attached, circular flap to just under Bowman's layer. The underlying stromal bed is then treated with the laser, and the cap is repositioned. This procedure, laser in situ keratomileusis (LASIK), is virtually painless and avoids the haze that might have occurred in Bowman's layer. It requires topical anesthesia and a special instrument for creating the flap.

Other procedures currently approved to correct refractive errors include 1) Intacs™ (Addition Technology, Des Planes, IL), a reversible insertion of curved plastic strips in the peripheral cornea, and 2) phakic IOLs, which are placed in front of the natural lens.

For more details on refractive procedures, please see the Series title *Refractive Surgery for Eyecare Paraprofessionals*.

Suture Adjustments

Once the major part of an ocular procedure has been done, the results can often be fine tuned by adjusting sutures during the postoperative period. Certain muscle recession procedures in strabismus surgery are specifically designed to allow an adjustment in the 24 hours following the operation to ensure ocular alignment and to maximize the potential for binocular fusion. Corneal procedures that require more than a few sutures, such as some cataract extractions or corneal transplantations, may be subject to induced astigmatism from the suturing. Adjustment of sutures can reduce this astigmatism. Both muscle and corneal suture adjustments can be done at the slit lamp with topical anesthetics.

Instruments

`OphA`
`Srg`

In the huge armamentarium of surgical instruments, there are only a few that are routinely used in minor ocular procedures. These are described below and shown in Figures 12-1 to 12-6.

Lid Speculum

The spring-loaded wire speculum or locking metal speculum is used to hold the upper and lower eyelids apart. Once inserted, these instruments remain in place. Individual lids may be held away from the surgical site by handheld retractors such as the Berens (Figure 12-1).

Scissors

There are many variations on the standard scissors style for ocular surgery (Figure 12-2). Blades may be curved or straight, short or long; tips may be sharp or blunt; the scissor may be closed with the standard side-by-side finger loops, or the closure may be accomplished by a

Figure 12-1. Holding instruments (retractors). (A) Stevenson lacrimal sac retractor. (B) Conway lid retractor. (C) Berens lid elevator. (D) Lid expressor. (E) Arruga glove retractor. (Reprinted from Jackson-Williams B. *Ophthalmic Surgical Assisting*. Thorofare, NJ: SLACK Incorporated; 1993.)

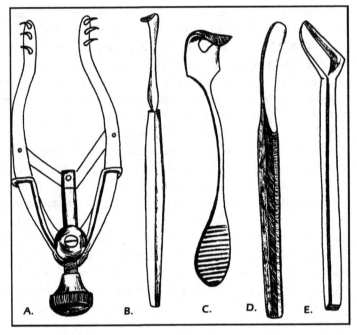

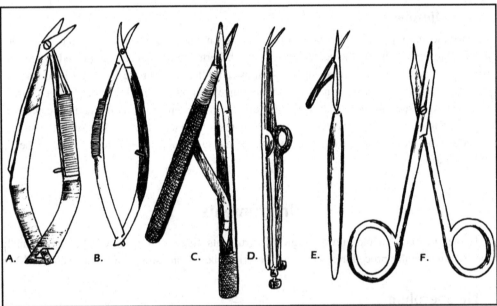

Figure 12-2. Cutting and working instruments: (A) Castroviejo corneoscleral punch. (B) Castroviejo corneal scissors. (C) Castroviejo blade breaker. (D) De Wecker's iridectomy scissors. (E) Moyes iridectomy scissors. (F) Stevens tenotomy scissors. (Reprinted from Jackson-Williams B. *Ophthalmic Surgical Assisting*. Thorofare, NJ: SLACK Incorporated; 1993.)

connected handle that acts like a spring. Some scissors are designed for very specific uses, such as cutting the corneal limbus.

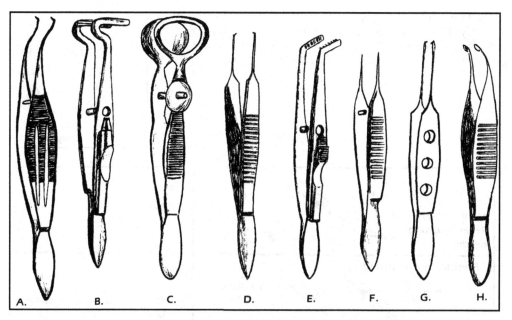

Figure 12-3. Holding instruments (forceps): (A) Hyde corneal. (B) Berke ptosis. (C) Des Marres chalazion. (D) Lester fixation. (E) Jameson muscle. (F) Dressing. (G) Bishop-Harmon. (H) Arruga capsule. (Reprinted from Jackson-Williams B. *Ophthalmic Surgical Assisting.* Thorofare, NJ: SLACK Incorporated; 1993.)

Forceps

This tweezerlike instrument is used for picking up or holding tissue (hence the pseudonym *pick-ups*). The opposing tips may be smooth, ridged for better gripping, or toothed to hold tissue securely. Forceps are manufactured in different sizes, and some can be locked in the closed position (Figure 12-3).

Needles/Sutures

Ocular surgery generally requires fine sutures and needles (Figure 12-4). The needles are curved and may have one or more cutting edges in addition to the point. Needles are manufactured with a variety of different shaped points. Sutures are made of various materials with different tensile strengths and thicknesses; some sutures remain in the tissue permanently, others are absorbed by the tissue. Sutures are packaged already attached to the blunt end of the needle. All needles must be accounted for at the end of a procedure.

Needleholders

Because the needles and sutures for ocular surgery are so fine and small, they cannot be manipulated by the hands alone. Needleholders are forceplike instruments that the surgeon uses to carry and guide the needle and suture through the tissue. These instruments have a locking mechanism to hold the needle securely.

Figure 12-4. (A) Needle components. (B) Ophthalmic needle points and body shapes with typical applications. (C) Ophthalmic needle body shapes. (Reprinted from Jackson-Williams B. *Ophthalmic Surgical Assisting.* Thorofare, NJ: SLACK Incorporated; 1993.)

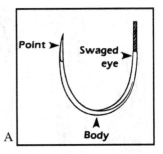

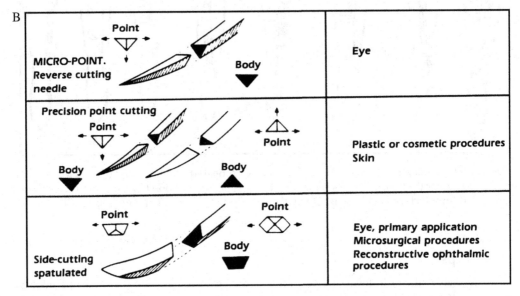

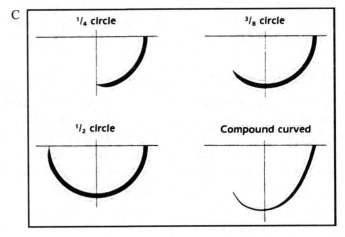

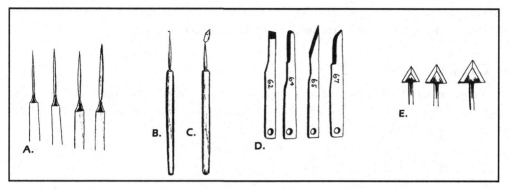

Figure 12-5. Cutting instruments: (A) Graefe cataract knives. (B) Castroviejo keratome. (C) Graefe Cystotome. (D) Beaver miniblades. (E) Jaeger keratomes. (Reprinted from Jackson-Williams B. *Ophthalmic Surgical Assisting*. Thorofare, NJ: SLACK Incorporated; 1993.)

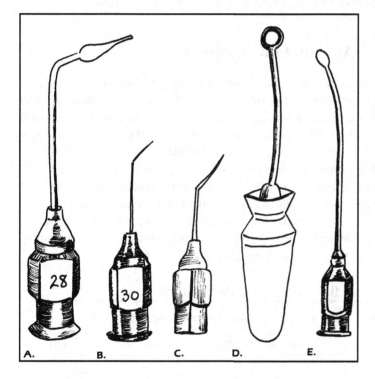

Figure 12-6. Working instruments (cannulas): (A) Tulevich lacrimal cannula. (B) Air injection cannula. (C) Cyclodialysis cannula. (D) Bell erisophake. (E) Troutman alpha chymotrypsin cannula. Note: Instruments are enlarged to show detail. (Reprinted from Jackson-Williams B. *Ophthalmic Surgical Assisting*. Thorofare, NJ: SLACK Incorporated; 1993.)

Scalpel/Knife

These cutting instruments are provided as a disposable blade and a separate blade holder (Figure 12-5). Blades come in different shapes with a standard configuration for attachment to the holder. A special knife has been developed for refractive surgery; it has a diamond blade that is extremely thin and sharp, and its carrier attaches to the handle.

Hemostat

Fashioned like standard scissors, this instrument grasps tissue like forceps. The hemostat has a ratcheted locking system that produces enough tissue compression to stop blood flow. Once locked in the closed position, the hemostat does not have to be held. This instrument may also be used to clamp drapes away from the surgical site or to clamp off tubing.

Cannula

This small metal tube is used to deliver liquids, such as balanced salt solution (BSS), to the surgical site. It looks like a thick needle with a blunt or olive-shaped tip and attaches to a bottle or syringe (Figure 12-6).

Cautery

This instrument has a wire tip that carries an electrical current and is used to seal blood vessels and stop blood flow. Its current is supplied either by a free-standing power box or, when less or nonvariable current is required, by a battery installed in the instrument itself. The cautery must always be checked for sufficient or appropriate power before the procedure begins.

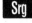

Assisting the Surgeon

The assistant is often the point person of the surgical arena, helping the surgeon to prepare and tending to the patient. Prior to beginning the surgical set-up, the assistant should be sure that the patient's questions and concerns have been addressed. The physician or a surgical counselor will have explained the procedure, its attendant risks and alternatives, and will have obtained the patient's signature on the informed consent form. See the Series title *Overview of Ocular Surgery and Surgical Counselling.* The patient may be very apprehensive; a calm, compassionate, and confident approach will often help allay his or her fears. An experienced, professional assistant will be able to answer any further questions the patient may have or defer them to the physician. Maintaining the patient's privacy and right to confidentiality are extremely important in the surgical setting, as the patient's apprehension may prompt personal disclosures that should not be communicated to anyone except the physician, if necessary.

What the Patient Needs to Know

- You have the right to expect a clean, neat, well-organized operating room.

- You should see evidence of instrument sterility, such as sealed packages, gloved personnel, etc.

- Let the surgeon or assistant know if you are uncomfortable or overly nervous.

- You must be relaxed enough to hold very still during the procedure.

- You have the right to information about your condition and its treatment.

In addition to tending to the patient, keeping a clean and sterile surgical environment, and maintaining instruments and equipment, the assistant is often called upon to directly assist the surgeon in the procedure. The assistant should do exactly and only what the surgeon requests. If the surgeon asks for a particular instrument, it is not up to the assistant to offer a similar but different one. The assistant may also be asked to hold tissue away from the surgical site, cut sutures,

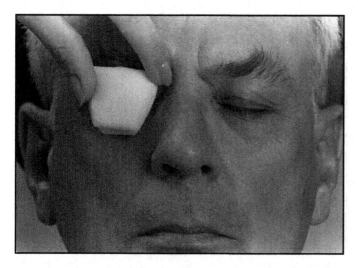

Figure 12-7. One eye pad is folded in half and placed under the eye pads if the patient has deep-set eyes. (Photo by Mark Arrigoni.) (Reprinted from Herrin MP. *Ophthalmic Examination and Basic Skills*. Thorofare, NJ: SLACK Incorporated; 1990.)

keep the surgical site clean or dry, etc. An experienced assistant will become familiar with each procedure and the surgeon's preferences in performing them and will be able to anticipate the need for particular instruments or assistance.

The assistant is responsible for having the proper fixatives available for tissue samples that are to be cultured or prepared for a pathology evaluation. Usually, the physician will handle tissue collection and any necessary prefixative preparation. However, if this task is delegated to the assistant, it is imperative that he or she know which fixatives or culture media are required. All samples must be labeled with the date, patient's name and record number, diagnosis, site from which the sample was taken, and the physician's name.

Dressings

Once a procedure has been completed, the assistant will clean the patient's face, instill whatever postoperative medications are indicated (usually an antibiotic and an anti-inflammatory drug), and apply a clean dressing to the eye. When a pressure patch is indicated, first fold a patch in half and position it over the closed lid (Figure 12-7). Then, place a second (unfolded) patch over the first. The unfolded pad is placed at a slight angle across the lid and taped firmly in place. Care must be taken that the tape does not extend into the hairline or interfere with the mouth (Figure 12-8). When a pressure patch is not necessary, a single open eye pad is applied as described.

Assisting With Laser Surgery

 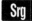

The advent of and rapid advances in laser technology have been a boon to clinical ophthalmology. The past 20 years have seen the use of lasers to treat retinal vascular problems, provide a noninvasive alternative to some glaucoma procedures, correct myopia, and treat both intraocular and external lesions. The light amplification by stimulated emission of radiation (LASER) is a powerful source of monochromatic light energy (ie, emitted at a particular wavelength of the electromagnetic spectrum). Different wavelengths of laser light are absorbed by different colored

Figure 12-8. Direct the tape away from the mouth. (Photo by Mark Arrigoni.) (Reprinted from Herrin MP. *Ophthalmic Examination and Basic Skills.* Thorofare, NJ: SLACK Incorporated; 1990.)

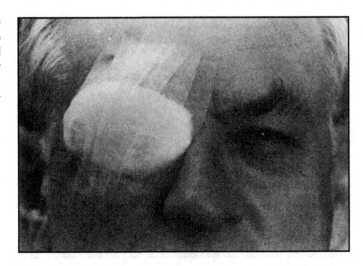

tissue (eg, hemoglobin or melanin), therefore, different lasers are used in different sites in the eye. The combination of laser type and tissue characteristics determines how the target tissue will be altered.

The blue-green light of the argon laser is used for blood coagulation or procedures requiring sealing of blood vessels. The longer wavelength of the krypton red laser allows deeper penetration of tissue. The CO_2 laser light is absorbed by water and is used in tissue with a high water content. All of these lasers alter tissue by thermal photocoagulation. Other types of lasers produce tissue damage by ionization (photodisruption) or photochemical changes. The neodymium: yttrium-aluminum-garnet (Nd:YAG) laser is an ionization type of instrument used to produce a hole in an opacified or thickened posterior lens capsule after cataract extraction. It may also be used to release intraocular cyclitic membranes. Very short wavelength (in the ultraviolet spectrum) lasers have been approved to ablate (destroy) anterior corneal tissue after scarring or for correcting refractive errors. These are the *excimer* lasers.

The assistant will primarily be in charge of preparing the patient, checking that the informed consent has been signed, and applying medications and/or dressings as needed. In addition, the assistant may be responsible for the day-to-day maintenance of one or more lasers in the office. It is important that the assistant either read the manual of operations for each laser or be trained by the manufacturer to perform only the simplest maneuvers (eg, turning the machine on and off). The physician is the only one credentialed to use the instrument.

Chapter 13

Patient Services

- Return patient calls promptly, and treat the patient with respect.

- Be sure that any information given to pharmacists or opticians is accurate and current.

- The patient is entitled to the information in his or her medical record.

- No information about a patient should be disclosed without his or her signed consent.

Scribing

The eyecare professional often serves the patient by assuming some of the chores in routine patient care. These duties may include acting as a scribe (ie, writing in the medical record what the physician says as he or she is examining the patient). Having a scribe allows the physician to devote full attention to the patient. While the doctor is performing the exam, he or she should relate the findings to the patient in layman's terms; the scribe records these findings in the medical record at the same time. This running commentary to the patient not only provides information but also helps the patient feel as though the doctor has spent more time with him or her. The scribe should write the diagnosis and note any detailed explanations given to the patient. Medications prescribed should be recorded in detail, including name, strength, dose, and whether these are additions or changes. It is important that this information be accurate and complete so that it can be easily accessed later, if necessary.

In addition to recording information, the scribe will also be available to help the doctor with the examination by holding the patient's lids, instilling drops, etc. Once the doctor has left the room, the scribe may remain to answer any questions, help the patient out of the chair, or direct the patient through the office to check out.

Patient Phone Calls

The assistant may also be asked to return patient telephone calls or to call in prescriptions to pharmacies or optical shops. Phone calls should be returned as soon as possible and with the patient's chart at hand. If the patient has a question about his or her treatment, it should be easy to provide this information if it has been properly recorded in the chart. However, if the patient has a question about his or her condition or new symptoms, the doctor should probably be consulted or asked to speak with the patient personally. Explain to the patient that "it is usually impossible to evaluate the condition of your eye over the phone, and you should be seen by the doctor." The doctor or assistant must then decide how urgent this situation might be and schedule the visit accordingly. All phone conversations should be documented in the patient's chart.

An experienced, knowledgeable assistant will be able to handle many questions called in to the office, but care must be taken that any information given is accurate and that the conversation is discreet. The patient has the right to speak with the physician if requested, and the assistant should never be afraid to defer a difficult, complicated, or sensitive question to the physician.

Prescriptions

When the assistant calls in or confirms either drug or optical prescriptions, accuracy is imperative. Prescriptions for either medicine or optical correction must be read exactly as the physician has written them. If there is any question or confusion about a prescription, it must be clarified by the physician before the information is relayed to the pharmacist or optician.

All prescriptions have 3 sections. The heading, usually preprinted, has the prescriber's name, address, and phone number. The patient's name, address, and phone number are written next, along with the date. The second section contains the prescription itself. The symbol *Rx* is written, followed by the name of the drug, its strength or concentration, and the amount to be dispensed. The directions to the patient indicate the amount of medication to be taken and how often.

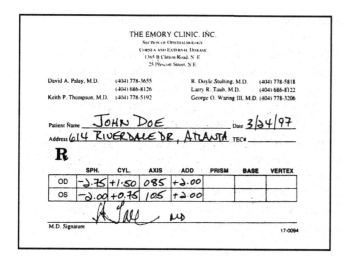

Figure 13-1. Spectacle prescription in plus cylinder form.

The third section of the form has the physician's signature, Drug Enforcement Administration (DEA) number, and refill instructions. Here is an example:

Rx   Pred Forte 0.1% ophthal soln

          disp 15 ml

          sig 1 gtt to OS QID

Common abbreviations used in medical prescriptions are listed in Table 1-1.

Attention to certain details of prescription writing will help avoid errors. Prescriptions should be written legibly in ink, using metric measures and avoiding uncommon abbreviations. There should be some record of the prescription in the chart, especially if it has been called in to the pharmacy. Cautionary instructions to the patient might include "may cause drowsiness," "for relief of pain," "finish all pills," etc.

For optical correction prescriptions, the heading is the same. The prescription section usually has a table with the top row for the right eye (OD) and the bottom row for the left eye (OS). The columns are for the sphere power, the cylinder power, the cylinder axis, the bifocal or trifocal add, and prism power, if indicated. The third section contains the doctor's signature and any special instructions to the optician.

A glasses prescription is always written in this order:

(+ or -) sphere (+ or -) cylinder x axis (001 - 180).

The sphere and cylinder powers are written out to the hundredth decimal place (eg, -2.75 +1.50 x 085). If the sphere power is zero, *plano* is written; if the cylinder power is zero, a line is drawn through the cylinder and axis spaces on the form. If any power is less than one, a zero is placed before the decimal (eg, 0.75) (Figure 13-1).

Patient Education

Another area for which the assistant may become responsible is patient education. Often, the office has preprinted literature on a variety of common ocular disorders and treatments. The assistant should become familiar with the contents of these brochures in order to accurately answer any questions that may arise about them. In addition, the physician may ask the patient to view a video that explains a planned procedure. The assistant should be available after the viewing to answer or refer questions to the physician.

Whenever the assistant has occasion to explain information to the patient, it should be done in simple language without talking down to the patient. For instance, medical terms such as sclera or strabismus can be replaced by the layman's terms *white of the eye* and *crossed eyes*. Often, patients will inquire about how much a procedure will hurt. It helps to calm the patient if the word *pain* is avoided. Instead, the assistant may say that there might be some *discomfort* but that operative anesthesia and postoperative analgesics will be used to minimize this.

Finally, the patient has the right to know the details of his or her condition and treatment and is entitled to the information in his or her medical record. The physical record is a legal document that is the property of the practice, but the information in it is the property of the patient. The record may be copied or summarized on the patient's written request or signed release. A telephone request is not sufficient; an actual signature must be obtained.

What the Patient Needs to Know

- The assistant who may help you is your doctor's trusted employee.

- You have the right to speak to the physician; your call will usually be returned as soon as it is convenient.

- If there is an emergency, tell the assistant and ask to speak to the doctor immediately.

- You have the right to privacy and discretion.

- Remember that the doctor is busy caring for other patients who have problems, too.

- Although your records belong to the office, you have the right to the information in them.

Index

Printed in the United States
by Baker & Taylor Publisher Services